T0208713

Also by Allen B. Weisse

Medicine: State of the Art
Conversations in Medicine
Medical Odysseys
The Man's Guide to Good Health
The Staff and the Serpent
Heart to Heart
Lessons in Mortality

Notes of a Medical Maverick

Allen B. Weisse, M.D.

iUniverse, Inc.
New York   Bloomington

Notes of a Medical Maverick

Copyright © 2010 by Allen B. Weisse, M.D.

All rights reserved. No part of this book may be used or reproduced by any means, graphic, electronic, or mechanical, including photocopying, recording, taping or by any information storage retrieval system without the written permission of the publisher except in the case of brief quotations embodied in critical articles and reviews.

iUniverse books may be ordered through booksellers or by contacting:

iUniverse
1663 Liberty Drive
Bloomington, IN 47403
www.iuniverse.com
1-800-Authors (1-800-288-4677)

Because of the dynamic nature of the Internet, any Web addresses or links contained in this book may have changed since publication and may no longer be valid. The views expressed in this work are solely those of the author and do not necessarily reflect the views of the publisher, and the publisher hereby disclaims any responsibility for them.

ISBN: 978-1-4502-5933-0 (sc)
ISBN: 978-1-4502-5935-4 (dj)
ISBN: 978-1-4502-5934-7 (ebook)

Library of Congress Control Number: 2010914031

Printed in the United States of America

iUniverse rev. date: 11/08/2010

To Danielle and Chick: two of the best ideas of any kind I ever had.

... my hope is in the love of truth and in the integrity of intelligence.

William Harvey, M.D.
Anatomical Studies on the Motion of the Heart and Blood (1628)

Contents

ACKNOWLEDGMENTS

Most of the material contained herein has not been previously published. Some of the essays have appeared in unaltered or slightly modified form in: *Hospital Practice* (In the Service of the IRS, Confessions of Creeping Obsolescence); *Pharos* (The Phoenix Phenomenon in Medical Research); *Journal of the History of Medicine and Allied Sciences* (The Elusive Clot); *The American Journal of Cardiology* (The First Heart Operation); *The Journal of Cardiac Failure* (A Fond Farewell to the Foxglove?); *Perspectives in Biology & Medicine* (I Was a Mole in an IRB); and *Baylor University Medical Center Proceedings* (Absolutely the Last Word on Physical Diagnosis. Not!).

For each chapter, where indicated, helpful reviewers have been identified. For the book as a whole I am indebted, as always, to my mate, my muse and my most cherished critic, Dr. Laura Weisse.

1

WHY "MAVERICK"?

IN MY OTHER LIFE, that of an academic cardiologist, I came to a fork in the road fairly early in the game. In 1963 I had just been appointed an instructor of medicine at the medical school where I would remain for the rest of my career and had to decide which professional path I would follow. To the left lay the path of super specialization; I could select a rather abstruse cardiovascular condition and devote myself unremittingly to it until I had a good chance of becoming one of the world experts on it. There was the risk, however, as some cynics might postulate, of getting to know more and more about less and less until I knew all there was to know about nothing at all. To the right lay the path of uncertainty; I could let my efforts wander in whatever direction my curiosity led them. Although I might have to settle on becoming a jack of all trades instead of a master of one, there was the compensation that "jacks," after all is said and done, might have a lot more fun than "masters."

I deliberately veered to the right and never really looked back. The expectation of never becoming a world class expert was certainly fulfilled, but I was rewarded with the opportunity to explore fields far beyond clinical and experimental cardiology while still maintaining credentials required for my day job as a member of our medical faculty. Ethics, philosophy and especially history, a great love of my life, were given free rein in my writings often flavored by large dollops of humor.

As a result of this, although many of my efforts fell into the conventional modes of medical publishing, others found it difficult to find a home within the pages of learned or even popular journals. If an article touched on an aspect of medical history the historical journals were more than likely to reject it. Oftentimes the reviewers would remark on its interest and literary quality, but the final judgment would be "not for us." Medical journals, cardiological and otherwise, would come up with the same decision. My penchant for humor was particularly self-defeating. Although laughter is supposed to have a healing quality, it rarely finds its way into serious repositories of professional medical writing. So it is that although some of the essays appearing here have previously been published in scholarly journals many of them have remained in limbo until appearing here for the first time.

The term "maverick" has been overused as of late, especially in politics in describing some of its practitioners and probably should be given a rest. However, it so neatly describes what I have often been about that I could not resist using it to describe what is contained within these pages.

You may be interested to learn that the term harks back to a living person. Samuel Augustus Maverick (1803-1870) was a Texas lawyer, politician and rancher who refused to brand his cattle, probably because he was not all that interested in this aspect of his life. The term "maverick" came to be used to describe the independently minded although I prefer to think of it more metaphorically; his cattle had no brand to mark them and therefore could not be identified or categorized as part of any group. Thus each retained its uniqueness and individuality.

Proceeding within this Western context of the term I look upon much of my work as *unbranded stock* that may wander far beyond the local *spread*. Since you, dear reader, have already gotten this far along the way I hope that your interests, like mine are far *ranging*. I trust that you will not be inclined to *ride off into the sunset* but choose rather to *saddle up* and join me on this *trail* of discovery, surprise, and inspiration enjoying an occasional chuckle along the way.

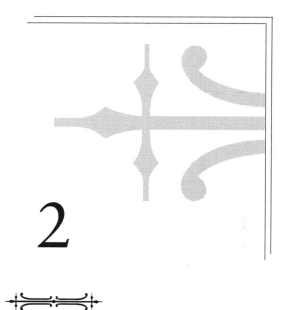

2

THE PHOENIX PHENOMENON IN MEDICAL RESEARCH

SOME YEARS AGO IT was suggested that "The Phoenix Phenomenon" might be a term suitably applied to ideas in science and medicine that, although presented as original concepts, actually had been proposed in the past, rejected and forgotten until now arising again like the mythical bird, the Phoenix, from its own ashes.[1] Some recent readings however suggested that this term might even be better applied to instances in which some investigator may have suffered some devastating loss – critical data, the ability to reproduce results, one's personal health or special knowledge – despite which he or she was able to overcome this debacle and move on to ultimately achieve the treasured final goal.

Stimulating this revised conception were retellings of two instances of this kind, one not actually involving medicine; the other more appropriately described as being within the general field of biology.

The first concerns the Scottish essayist and historian Thomas Carlyle (1795-1881) and the writing of his masterpiece, a history of the French Revolution (1837), which established him as a major figure in Victorian England. An intriguing aspect of this massive effort concerns its near derailment at an early stage in its production.[2]

When Carlyle had completed a draft of the first volume of what would become a three volume account of the events leading up to, occurring during and then at the end of the great political conflagration across the Channel, he turned the manuscript over to his good friend John Stuart Mill for comments and suggestions. In March of 1835 Mill appeared at Carlyle's home overcome

7

with grief and remorse. Somehow Mill's housekeeper had mistaken the manuscript for wastepaper and only a few charred pages had survived the fireplace. One can only imagine the anguish that this most assuredly must have caused in Carlyle, but to his everlasting credit he was able to overcome his own feelings of despair in order to comfort his friend. A letter followed in which Carlyle wrote "You left me last night with a look which I shall not soon forget. Is there anything that I could do or suffer or say to alleviate you? For I feel that your sorrow must be far sharper than mine...Courage, my Friend."

Although in later years their friendship would suffer because of differences in philosophical and social outlooks, the magnanimity of Carlyle under these trying circumstances was never forgotten by Mill. Although Carlyle at first despaired of ever being able to recreate this beginning of the great work, following the completion of the second and third volumes of the trilogy he managed to turn back to the first and accomplish its rewriting.

Closer to the field of medicine was the career of Alfred Russel Wallace (1823-1913). It was an early incident in his long life that merits inclusion here. Wallace, it might be remembered, was the naturalist who came in second to Charles Darwin in recognition for the theory of natural selection (i.e. evolution). Wallace, after considering the subject for some years, solidified his beliefs about all this during a sojourn through the Malay Archipelago from 1854 to 1862. It was his early reports from this expedition and correspondence with Darwin about them that finally galvanized the latter into publishing *The Origin of Species* in 1859. Although the contributions of both men were acknowledged at a meeting of the Royal Society in 1858, it was Darwin who received primary recognition. Wallace was apparently grateful just to be mentioned at all given Darwin's high social and professional status at the time in contrast to his own penurious upbringing and checkered employment background up to that point.

In the present context it was an earlier episode in the long career of Wallace that was so striking as a reflection of his indomitable will.[3] Having begun some efforts as a naturalist in England, obtaining biological specimens for interested collectors, Wallace, at the age of 25, took off in 1848 for a four year trip to Brazil and up the Amazon to explore the Rio Negro and collect samples from the plethora of exotic natural specimens that awaited him there. After these years during which he suffered from various fevers, disabling physical injuries, near starvation at times and even the loss of a brother to yellow fever, Wallace left Brazil in 1852 with sixteen crates containing perhaps hundreds of preserved specimens and dozens of live birds and monkeys along with copious notes describing his discoveries. Unfortunately the ship that contained both him and his hard won cargo caught fire and all was lost to Wallace with the exception of a few of his notes. After ten days in an open lifeboat Wallace was rescued but "Four years of work dropped away like a cinder in a barrel."

Such a personal tragedy might have deterred another person from persisting along a path that had rewarded him only with hardship and failure. However Wallace, thanks to a small insurance policy on the cargo, was able to keep himself going for over a year upon his return to England and then, undeterred, embark on that trip to the Malay Archipelago where his evolutionary theories took final form.

In the light of these heroic episodes in the lives of Carlyle and Wallace it was tempting to seek similar demonstrations of resilience among pioneers in the field of medicine. Even within the experience of a single medical historian they have been found to be a not uncommon component to such careers.

Reminiscent of the Carlyle story concerning the loss of his early manuscript is an incident involving cardiologist Eugene Lepeschkin (1914-1994). Born in Russia, the son of a distinguished professor of plant physiology, Lepeschkin's early years were notably peripatetic as his father relocated from one academic appointment to another in Europe and the United States. Living in Arizona from 1927 to 1932 Lepeschkin actually graduated from high school in Tucson. However, when it was decided that Eugene was headed for a career in medicine his father took the family back to Europe so that his son might benefit from a medical education in the leading medical center of the time, Vienna.

At the outbreak of World War II, therefore, Lepeschkin was trapped in Europe and unable to obtain permission to return to the United States. Finding himself in a state of limbo in 1939 upon graduating from medical school, he devoted himself to compiling an all-inclusive monograph on the electrocardiogram. This was published in 1941 in German as *Das Elektrokardiogram*. It was not until 1947 when, invited by Dr. Wilhelm Raab to join the medical faculty at the University of Vermont that Lepeschkin was able to return to America. In the years between the publication of his German tome and his arrival in the States Lepeschkin had continued to collect thousands of new publications flooding the medical literature on the increasing use of electrocardiography in clinical medicine. These were all to be included in an updating of his text, now to be printed in English. What happened can best be described in his own words.[4]

"I had prepared the translation of my German book soon after arriving in the U.S. but had in the meantime been making so many additions and corrections that I did not want to have the manuscript typed until all the corrections were finished. Accordingly, when it became necessary for me to take the manuscript to the prospective publisher in Baltimore for clarification of certain points I took with me the only copy I had. On the way through New

York City I stopped at the residence of Dr. Bruno Kisch on the West Side to discuss some of his papers, and while I was talking to him someone broke into my car and stole the entire briefcase with the manuscript. I advertised in all the N.Y. papers offering a reward, but to no avail. I therefore had to rewrite the entire book, but in the process it became a much better work."

For those who think this might not have involved a major effort consider that *Das Elektrokardiogram* had 400 pages and 4000 references while *Modern Electrocardiography* published 10 years later in 1951 had 600 pages and nearly 10,000 references.[5]

Vital elements other than accumulated papers concerning research can be lost; such as the loss of a critical formula or technique. Consider James B. Collip (1892-1965) and the discovery of insulin.[6] At the end of 1921 Canadian surgeon Frederick Banting and his medical student assistant Charles H. Best were working under Prof. J.J.R. Macleod at the University of Toronto, attempting to isolate and purify insulin from beef pancreas for the treatment of diabetes. Since these two lacked the biochemical expertise needed to succeed in this attempt Macleod assigned Collip, a young physiologist and biochemist, to assist them. Collip had already established himself as a skillful and resourceful individual in his field and was rapidly advancing through the academic ranks. Collip did not disappoint; in about a month or so he succeeded in purifying the insulin obtained from the beef extracts. Soon after, with the cooperation of Connaught Laboratories, they planned to mass produce the hormone in Toronto to meet the urgent requests of clinicians throughout Canada and the United States who had learned of their efforts.

Just as production was about to begin Collip found that he could no longer produce the purified insulin that had been the result of his earlier efforts. Somehow or other he had simply lost the knack. The strain this produced for all four individuals can only be imagined and most severely in Collip who would nevertheless not give up but rather frantically persisted in trying to reproduce his earlier results with multiple variations in laboratory technique, some of these suggested in consultation with the other principals. Providentially Collip succeeded after several more weeks of effort and the rest, as they say, is (medical) history.

In 1923 the Nobel Prize in Medicine or Physiology was awarded to Banting and Macleod, a story in itself with a major brouhaha ensuing in which Banting publicly challenged the decision by giving half of his reward money to Best. Macleod responded in kind with a similar gesture to Collip. Whatever the controversy surrounding the full extent of Collip's role in the affair, he became a major figure in Canadian science, often looked upon as the father of Canadian endocrinology with a long and successful career to prove it.

Loss of technique is one thing, loss of "data" still another.

For many years it had been known that dietary deficiency could cause heart disease with heart failure related to severe thiamine deprivation (beri-beri) a prime example. It was also recognized that some alcoholic individuals, who often suffered multiple dietary deficiencies could occasionally develop heart muscle disease (cardiomyopathy). What was undetermined was whether these patients who developed heart disease did so because of the lack in their diet of essential nutritional factors or as a result of a toxic effect of the alcohol itself.

Timothy J. Regan (1924-2001) was keenly interested in this problem and for many years was chief of the cardiology division at the Seton Hall School of Medicine, (later the New Jersey Medical School) in Jersey City, New Jersey. It was there that he began his early studies on alcohol. One of his approaches to the problem was to develop in dogs a model in which the dietary element and the possible effects of alcohol could be separated. This involved maintaining a cohort of dogs with carefully determined adequate nutritional components in their diet as controls and another group that received all the necessary dietary supplements but whose total caloric makeup was altered to include ample amounts of alcohol, similar to those reported in alcoholic patients.

Modern animal facilities were not a high priority back in the 1950's through the early 1970s especially at a new school struggling to establish itself in Jersey City. Fortuitously, however, on the top floor of one of the three towers that constituted the Jersey City Medical Center there was space available for animal quarters. Despite the unusual location and its lack of conventional animal care amenities Regan took pains to keep his dogs well cared for including adequate heat in the winter and air conditioning during the summer.

Since it may take many years for cirrhosis of the liver, heart disease and other end-points of chronic alcoholism in humans to manifest themselves the dietary conditioning of Regan's dogs involved as many as 22 months. However, over one beastly hot summer weekend the air conditioning in the animal quarters failed and almost all of Regan's dogs perished. When I met him the following Monday I was prepared to find him in the depths of despair after such a loss. "What will you do now, Tim?" I asked. He smiled, "Get some more dogs, I guess." As a result he was finally able to demonstrate in the animal model both hemodynamic and histological effects of alcohol upon the heart.[7] These findings, along with the reports of studies involving humans from Regan's laboratory and others firmly established alcohol as a toxic agent for the heart as well as liver and central nervous system among patients addicted to its use.

Some years earlier a similar impasse confronted Alfred M. Prince (1928-)

who was called up for Army Service during the Korean War in 1959.[8] Without any previous experience in the field he was assigned to work on the problem of hepatitis that was affecting both American and Korean soldiers in the Far East. In 1962 with a colleague, Richard K. Gershon, he began a survey of 2500 soldiers collecting serum transaminase levels (a rise occurring with liver injury). By putting together the blood findings with the appearances of liver biopsies obtained from the abnormals they established evidence for a condition they called "chronic active hepatitis." Later, based now in Tokyo, Prince, on a visit to a Japanese army hospital, learned that of those who had received blood transfusions a full two-thirds had come down with hepatitis. This was something he felt he had to study.

With Gershon he collected sera and liver biopsies from nearly 60 patients. The collection was sent back for later study to Yale, Prince's home base in the United States. They were stored in a freezer in the pathology laboratories. Some months later Prince, who had now taken up a position at the Wistar Institute at the University of Pennsylvania in Philadelphia freed himself of his duties there in order to rush to New Haven to begin work on the specimens he and Gershon had so carefully collected. When they opened the old freezer the first thing to greet them was the rotting leg of a deer covered with maggots. To their horror they realized that the freezer had been out of commission for at least a few months. As for the specimens so painstakingly accumulated, what the heat had not destroyed had been finished off by the hydrochloric acid fumes from a tissue dissolving experiment being conducted by a professor of pathology. It could all have ended there. It didn't.

Sickened by this terrible disappointment but still undeterred, Prince decided to undertake a different type of prospective study in the United States but was turned down by both the University of Pennsylvania and Yale. However Prince finally found a home for this work, the New York Blood Center, where he embarked on further studies, ultimately cooperating with Baruch Blumberg on research regarding the pathogenesis of hepatitis. Blumberg would later receive the Nobel Prize in Medicine and Physiology for "discoveries concerning new mechanisms for the origin and dissemination of infectious diseases" no doubt aided and abetted in part by Prince's dogged enthusiasm.

In 2001 during a weekend of flooding in laboratories belonging to the Texas Medical Center of Baylor Medical School in Houston more than 30,000 research animals lost their lives. According to the Houston Chronicle this "… wiped out millions of dollars of federally funded research. Meticulously kept computer data were fried into electronic oblivion. And some students lost years' worth of their doctorate work." How many stories of defeat and triumph might well have arisen from the aftermath?

Of all the disastrous losses that might beset a medical investigator none is more crushing than the loss of a patient. The loss of a series of patients one is trying to help can only be considered incalculable. Willem J. Kolff (1911-2009) the Dutch physician who developed the first successful artificial kidney lost fourteen of the first fifteen patients he subjected to this treatment between 1943 and 1944.[9] This took a tremendous toll on Kolff but in his case, however, the blow might have been softened by the realization that the patients were in the final stages of acute or chronic renal failure with certain death only a few days distant at most. For those such as cardiac surgeons involved with the introduction of new, potentially dangerous new procedures the prognosis without surgery, although certainly grim, might be difficult to place in the future.

The history of surgery for mitral stenosis, the first successful direct operation upon the heart for cardiac disease, provides a paradigm in this regard. However this approach to treatment advanced only in fits and starts. Following multiple attempts in the 1920s by Elliott Carr Cutler, Samuel A. Levine and Claude S. Beck that ultimately failed the field remained fallow until the 1940s when at four separate sites surgeons felt justified in returning to the problem. Dwight E. Harken at Harvard's Peter Bent Brigham Hospital, Russell C. Brock at Guy's Hospital in London and Horace G. Smithy at the Medical College of South Carolina in Charleston were all, to a great extent, insulated from outside disapproval and pressures by the august institutions with which they were affiliated. The fourth member of this quadrumvirate, Charles P. Bailey (1910-1993) a flamboyant and free wheeling New Jersey surgeon who seemed to operate beyond the bounds of any one institution, proved a more accessible target for his detractors. As he moved ahead with his surgical approach to open up the narrowed mitral valve he found himself increasingly isolated and at risk for losing all of his operating privileges at the hospitals to which he had been affiliated. What kept him going? Perhaps it was the memory of his own father coughing up blood while in the final throes of his own losing battle against mitral stenosis or was it something else within Bailey's psychological makeup? Perhaps the feelings of many in similar positions were mirrored in Bailey's own words about his predicament[10]:

"Finally, however, you have to face the 'moment of truth' and the poignancy is so great that I can't really express it. You know that almost all the world is against you; you know that you have a great personal stake and might even lose your medical license, or at least your hospital privileges if you persist. In fact, the thought crosses your mind that maybe you really *are* crazy. And yet you feel that it has to be done and it must be right."

At a later period in the history of cardiac surgery, following John H. Gibbon, Jr.'s initial success on closing an atrial septal defect using his heart-lung machine in 1953, he had multiple failures and made no further attempts at this. There were other scattered individual attempts with heart-lung machines to correct congenital cardiac defects with no clear evidence of the efficacy of this approach demonstrated. In response to this state of affairs John W. Kirklin (1917-2004), then at the Mayo Clinic in Minnesota, determined to perform a series of such procedures. Eight patients were brought to surgery; four died following the procedure.[11] Despite the high mortality this was taken as an indication of success rather than failure and open heart surgery was on its way. Those who might have considered Kirklin callous in ignoring the children that had perished at his hands might be interested to learn that the laconic Kirklin – who rarely expressed his feelings publicly – was known to disappear for a day or two following the loss of a patient in order to collect himself and then move on.

Loss of self, mental or physical, can also represent a catastrophic event for a physician. Early in his career as a surgeon and later medical writer and historian Sherwin B. Nuland (1930-) suffered a depression so severe that it required his admission to a mental hospital. No medications or psychotherapy seemed to have any effects and lobotomy was being considered. Then, somehow, Nuland found the strength to reach within in order to deliver himself from the abyss through sheer will power.[12] Despite a few minor recurrences of the depression a remarkably productive career has followed.

No less damaging and much longer lasting was the physical damage suffered by Arthur C. Guyton (1919-2003) when, in 1946, he was struck down by poliomyelitis while working as a surgical resident toward a career as a cardiac surgeon at Massachusetts General Hospital in Boston.[13] The resulting paralysis affected almost his entire body at first and even after months of rehabilitation he still had total paralysis of the left shoulder and arm as well as the right leg. These deficiencies along with severe weakness of the right shoulder and remaining extremities would remain with him for the rest of his life. He would be confined to a wheel chair for the duration.

At the time Guyton was married and already starting a family. With his hopes for a career in surgery or any other source of gainful employment seemingly doomed, he was moved with his family back to his home in Oxford, Mississippi. But Guyton, even this early in his career, had already demonstrated his research ability both as an undergraduate at "Ole Miss" and in medical school at Harvard. In 1947 this led to his appointment in the pharmacology department at the University of Mississippi with a part time position with the department of physiology. At about that time an opening for the position of departmental head in physiology unexpectedly occurred. Guyton, who was already a recipient of a N.I.H. grant to study pulmonary edema was given a trial at the post. After 20 months Guyton was appointed permanently as chairman and remained there for the next 41 years, a record for such a position. During this time he established himself as a brilliant investigator of the circulation and as one of the great teachers of physiology primarily through his textbook which was updated every five years from the first edition (1956) and authored solely by Guyton until the ninth edition in 1996. It has been translated into 15 languages and distributed all over the world. The royalties from this helped fund the medical education of his ten children who all followed in his career choice of medicine. What the world lost in what certainly would have been a brilliant cardiac surgeon it gained in one of the great physiology researcher-teachers of all time.

One popular view of the medical researcher is that of a lonely individual quietly tolling away behind closed laboratory doors, struggling with problems over the years but making steady progress finally to emerge with his chosen goal. In many instances this may be true, but in others the work is carried on in the public arena. The problems that may arise can include the serious and even the catastrophic. The ability of some remarkable individuals to recover from such appalling setbacks can well be considered Phoenix-like in character.

REFERENCES:

1. Weisse AB. *Medical Odysseys. The Different and Sometimes Unexpected Pathways to Medical Discoveries.* New Brunswick:Rutgers Univ. Press, 1991; 2-3.

2. Cohen R. Can You Forgive Him? *The New Yorker,* Nov. 8, 2004:48-65.

3. Quammen D. *The Reluctant Mr. Darwin. An Intimate Portrait of Charles Darwin and the Making of His Theory of Evolution.* New York:Norton, 2006:122-132.

4. Lepeschkin E. Letter to A.B. Weisse, Oct. 16, 1990.

5. Lepeschkin E. *Modern Electrocardiograpy.* Baltimore:Williams & Wilkins, 1951.

6. Bliss M. *The Discovery of Insulin.* Chicago:Univ. of Chicago Press, 1982:129-134.

7. Regan TJ, Khan MI, Ettinger PO, Haider B, Lyons MM, Oldewurtel HA. Myocardial function and lipid metabolism in the chronic alcoholic animal. *J Clin Invest* 1974; 54:740-745.

8. Weisse AB. *Medical Odysseys:* 25-28.

9. Kolff WJ in Weisse AB. *Conversations in Medicine. The Story of Twentieth-Century American Medicine in the Words of Those Who Created It.* New York: New York Univ. Press, 1984:354

10. Bailey CP in Weisse AB. *Conversations in Medicine*: 136-141.

11. Kirklin JW, DuShane JW, Patrick RT, Donald DE, Hetzel PS, Wood EH. Intracardiac surgery with the aid of a mechanical pump-oxygenator system (Gibbon type). Report of eight cases. *Proc Staff Meet Mayo Clinic* 1955; 30:201-206.

12. Nuland SB. *Lost in America. A Journey With My Father.* New York:Alfred Knopf, 2003:4-9.

13. Guyton AC in Weisse AB. *Heart to Heart. The Twentieth-Century Battle Against Cardiac Disease. An Oral History.* New Brunswick:Rutgers Univ. Press, 2002:120-124.

3

IN THE SERVICE OF THE IRS

LIKE ANY OTHER RED blooded American, I want as little to do with the Internal Revenue Service as is humanly possible. But when this arm of our government calls for your help in retrieving multi-millions of dollars that some nefarious plotters have excluded from our dwindling treasury, who can resist this appeal to patriotism? Certainly not I, and when the call came to me, I was soon knee deep in the controversy surrounding the alleged scam.

The genesis of the case was actually more than two world wars ago. Shortly before the outbreak of hostilities between the United States and Germany in World War I, a major German industrial giant, fearful of having its substantial American holdings confiscated , turned them all over to an employee who was a faithful American national but who, in the final analysis, could also be relied upon to do his duty for the parent company. At the conclusion of the war in 1918 when these holdings were turned back to the German company, their American agent was rewarded for his stalwart performance with large chunks of stock, the basis for his family's fortune.

The only son and heir of this man was as astute and hard working as his father, and managed to increase the family's wealth even more, aided in part by the effect of economic trends over the next thirty or forty years. As he continued to amass this enormous wealth he waited until middle age before acquiring someone to share it with him, oddly enough a simple American farm girl, far removed from the opulent kind of existence that had always surrounded her husband. This down home direct approach to life, unaffected by all the trappings of wealth, never deserted her and was a distinct part of her charm and attraction as she filled her husband's home with several children before he passed on many years before her.

As the sole heir to the fortune upon the death of her husband, the youngish widow never remarried but instead devoted herself to her children and grandchildren for the many remaining years of her life. It was an uninterrupted robust one until her early seventies when she developed a serious condition of one of her heart valves, aortic stenosis. It soon became necessary for open heart surgery to be undertaken and the diseased valve was replaced with a mechanical prosthesis.

Soon after the successful surgery, she began to divest herself of large portions of her wealth, transferring it to her daughters and sons who were now in their forties and fifties and already with children of their own entered into adulthood. By the time the elderly lady finally did succumb to her heart disease seven years post surgery, all but a fraction of her former fortune was now in the hands of her surviving children.

The U.S. government's contention was that this transfer of wealth on the part of the widow was a deliberate scheme to avoid estate taxes in the face of her realization that only a few years of life would be left to her following such a major operation in a person of her advanced age. The family's defense against this charge was that their mother and grandmother had no anticipation at all of dying so soon after her successful heart surgery. Aside from the valve problem her health had always been unusually good. The surgery and its aftermath had gone smoothly and all the symptoms that had precipitated the need for surgery in the first place had disappeared rapidly postoperatively. Her own mother had lived until the age of 96 and her family indicated that the old lady at their head, following replacement of the defective valve, had every intention of doing the same if not even bettering the record.

The reason for her breaking up the family fortune, they maintained, was that she realized late in life that even if she was to live until the age of 106 she could never manage to spend a significant portion of her money even if she was shamefully extravagant, something which she certainly was not.. Her intention in distributing her wealth when she did was to enable her children and grandchildren to enjoy it at a time in life when their own health was good and they could most enjoy the advantages of the kind of life style that this money could provide.

Therefore, basically it was not the state of her heart that was in question, but the state of her mind as she redistributed her wealth among her progeny. So where did I come in? As an expert in cardiovascular disease, I had the job of convincing the judge that life expectancy following such surgery in an elderly person was not great and thereby support the contention of the IRS that it was to avoid taxes that the disbursement of all these funds took place at this time during the matriarch's life.

On purely scientific grounds my medical case was easily made. No matter how skillful the cardiac surgeon might be, the artificial heart valves of the time were far from ideal substitutes for our God-given natural valves. They were foreign bodies that we were inserting and they had moving parts that could become stuck. After thousands upon thousands of heart beats they could break free from the moorings to which they were sutured. Blood clots tended to form on their surfaces. These or excessive scar formation over the valve surface could result in obstruction. Finally, bacteria which are frequently released into our blood stream after dental manipulations or even vigorous tooth brushing but are routinely removed from the blood stream in normal individuals could often find a nesting site on such artificial valves and result in life threatening infections (prosthetic valve endocarditis).

All in all, it was estimated in one report that within five years of such valve insertions it was likely that in fifty percent of such patients one of these devastating complications might occur resulting in the need for risky re-operation if not the death of the patient. It was one of these complications that took the widow off so suddenly and unexpectedly.

The case was to be decided by a judge rather than jury and prior to the court date I met with the IRS lawyer with whom I was to prepare our presentation. The young man who visited my office immediately struck me by his close resemblance to Harvard's Alan Dershowitz but, I was soon to learn, the resemblance stopped there. Several weeks later we sat together in the courtroom having arrived a bit early to await the entrance of the opposition.

The doors at the rear of the courtroom swung open and a phalanx of very impressive lawyers from one of the most prestigious firms in the city ceremoniously made their way down the center aisle. To say they were impressive was an understatement. Majestic came to mind, and I cocked an ear, almost expecting to hear organ music accompanying the procession. They literally gleamed in confidence and sartorial splendor. I would have ventured a guess that even their shoelaces would have outpriced the entire wardrobe of the two government representatives opposing them. Following close behind their legal champions were the family imperial, with righteous indignation inscribed on each and every countenance.

The cardiologist they had employed to represent them was a very competent one who had cared for the deceased during her final years. Not surprisingly, he was himself descended from the higher reaches of society, he and his father before him having ministered to their needs over many decades. His role was simply to testify that, in his opinion, his patient had done extraordinarily well post-operatively, that her death had come as something of a surprise to him in view of her excellent response to surgery, and that, despite this, she had never indicated to him in any way that she had expected anything other than a great number of years left to her following her surgical ordeal.

The medical portion of the testimony was pretty straightforward. It was on the legal side that I was sure the government's case had faltered, in no small measure, I ascertained, due to the demeanor of its legal representative. My partner was well prepared but much too tentative. He did not speak up clearly and constantly seemed obliged to refer to his notes even though I knew he had committed them to memory. In short, it was not a stellar courtroom performance.

The opposition, on the other hand, was equally well prepared but silky smooth and bursting with confidence in their convictions. Endless depositions, affidavits and what-all were extracted from their gleaming attaché cases as they serenely laid their case before the judge. They were so adept and full of themselves that I wondered as an almost neutral observer if this might prove off-putting to the stern and laconic jurist who presided over the whole affair. For my part, I had no idea what had been in the old lady's mind as she doled out all those millions. I could easily have been persuaded that it really was the simple generosity of a loving mother and grandmother that motivated her actions in the final years of her life. Fortunately, it was not my case to decide.

The formal court presentations came to a close and the court retired to consider the evidence. The judgment rendered a week or so later, was that there were insufficient grounds to indicate that the woman had expected a foreshortened existence and thus the case was decided in favor of the family.

This did not, however, conclude my connection with the case. The judge's decision proved, on the contrary, only a stopping point along the road I was to travel with the IRS over the next year. My extended involvement with that agency hinged simply upon the fact that they seemed totally incapable of providing me with the fee specified when I agreed to testify for them.

It was not a lot of money, considering the amount of time and effort I expended, only a thousand dollars. Indeed, when I finally became aware that the sum hoped to be recovered by the government might run as high as thirteen million dollars, I calculated that, had they succeeded, my "cut" would have amounted to less than eight thousandths of one percent. Given my sense of civic duty, I could live with this even though the realization that the opposing lawyers and their doctor must have walked off with infinitely more could have poured salt into the wound if I chose to let it. It was the action, or rather inaction of the IRS that accomplished just this.

Three months went by with no check in the mail. I then began a round of telephone calls and correspondence to the various arms of the IRS that might have been involved, all to no avail. By the time nine months had elapsed after the decision had been handed down and I had still not been paid, I took the only other course left to me, an appeal to my congressman. He excelled at this sort of service for his constituents and a week after my appeal his office wrote me that they would get on my case. A week after this a check for one thousand dollars arrived from the IRS. A week later a second check for one thousand dollars arrived from the IRS.

After all the grief they had caused me, I was momentarily tempted to pocket the second check and just sit tight. Then an idea occurred to me as to how I might take one small step in the name of all those who had ever had to tangle with the IRS bureaucracy and one giant step for my own sense of self satisfaction and fun.

I cashed the second check and issued one of my own for $910 payable to the IRS. The practice of the agency was to charge a 12 percent annual rate of interest for all money owed them and vice versa if they, perchance, had owed any money to a taxpayer. Since this amounted to a monthly charge of one percent on any balance, I calculated that over nine months 90 dollars in interest had accrued to me. When I sent that check to the IRS little did I imagine how this was to shake the U.S. treasury to its very foundations. A flurry of telephone calls and correspondence followed in its wake all protesting that since the contract I had signed was only for $1000 and not $1090, there was no possible way that the system could tolerate such a deviation.

I was unmoved by such protestations. I knew very well that every day the IRS was breaking an assumed contract - the tax code - by making all kinds of deals with defaulting screen stars, sports heroes and Wall Street traders. Hundreds of thousands of dollars in taxpayer money had been written off in this way not to mention the hundreds of millions we have lost in the past to such deadbeats as Brazil and Poland, for example. In view of all this I refused to believe that my $90 represented an insurmountable obstacle to the survival of the system.

Finally the kid gloves came off and I began to receive calls and letters of a different nature. These all hinted darkly as to the possible role of the Department of Justice in my case if I did not come around. I actually warmed to the prospect of such an encounter and looked forward to the opportunity of revealing in open court how all those long distance telephone calls to me had probably already greatly exceeded the amount that they intended to recover in the first place. The time spent by secretaries and stenographers was an add on, not even to mention the hours of wasted attorneys' time spent in pursuit of my $90. By the time the threats had begun to arrive, all those phone calls had put me and the IRS attorney who was constantly in touch with me on an almost chummy basis. I verbalized about the possibilities of my testimony and how some magazines and talk show hosts might be interested in discussing how the government's money was routinely spent in such efforts.

As I began, almost palpably, to sense a rising discomfort at the other end of the line, I played my final card. To put an end to the business once and for all, as a gesture of good faith I would be willing to send a token sum to the IRS in settlement: $5.00. With visions of media mayhem probably dancing in his head, the lawyer replied that he would take it under advisement. A few days later his reply arrived.

"We have considered your gesture of conciliation," he wrote. "While the amount offered is not nearly as much as we had hoped, we have decided to accept your offer in the spirit in which it is made...When we receive your check we will close our file on the case."

And they did.

This all happened many years ago and I therefore am not concerned about ruffling the feathers of any individuals within the IRS by revealing it. My erstwhile adversaries have probably risen within the ranks and acquired enough mellowness to look upon this little imbroglio with almost as much amusement as I. It is equally as likely that, armed with all that knowledge about the inner workings of the IRS, they have even "deserted to the enemy" and proved invaluable within the ranks of accounting and law firms devoted to protecting other family fortunes from what they might consider unjustified depredations by the U.S. government.

Still there was some trepidation on my part in putting this all down in print for anyone to see. The IRS does not shine too brightly in the reflection of the light I have chosen to cast upon it and, deserved or not, it does have a reputation for vindictiveness. We are even aware that some previous administrations have used it to settle scores with offensive or offending individuals. But this is all in the past and could never be repeated in the present.

You might ask, "What, never?"

Well, hardly ever.

4

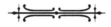

THE ELUSIVE CLOT: THE CONTROVERSY OVER CORONARY THROMBOSIS IN MYOCARDIAL INFARCTION

IN THE YEARS FOLLOWING World War II a growing spirit of elation began to spread among the medical community. It seemed, for a time, that the era of epidemic infectious disease was coming to an end. With the discovery of penicillin, streptomycin and other antibiotics a number of bacterial diseases could now be treated. Even tuberculosis, the "great white plague" could be cured in some patients. Improved and newly developed vaccines became available to prevent a number of viral diseases. In developed countries such as the United States the scourge of summertime, paralytic polio, would become a thing of the past and even the more deadly disease of smallpox would be completely eliminated by vaccination programs conducted by the World Health Organization.

Such wishful thinking about epidemic infectious disease would later be dispelled by the emergence of HIV and AIDS. But much before this, a different type of epidemic began to take hold in developed countries such as the United States and Western Europe. In the late 1940s and 1950s large numbers of individuals, mainly men in the prime of life, were succumbing to acute coronary occlusions. In some, sudden death occurred due to complete stoppage of the heart beat (asystole); in others a lethal irregularity of the heart contraction in which the normal beat was dispersed into multiple ineffective and uncoordinated contractions throughout the heart muscle (ventricular fibrillation) would have the same effect: an inability to pump blood out of the heart with the same mortal result. In patients who managed to survive the acute event without the occurrence of such lethal arrhythmias various amounts of heart muscle formerly supplied by the obstructed artery would be damaged (myocardial infarction). When extensive, either due to the single event or subsequent coronary occlusions, myocardial infarctions could result in diminished cardiac output with clinical heart failure developing and ultimately resulting in death weeks, months or occasionally years later. Among survivors, upon physical exertion requiring additional coronary flow, those areas of the heart supplied by partially obstructed arteries might become ischemic (lacking sufficient oxygen containing blood) and result in the symptom of chest pain or angina.

The recognition of predisposing factors to coronary occlusions, which would later be called risk factors, was in its infancy. Family history, smoking, hypertension, obesity, lipid abnormalities, diabetes could all play a role. But what was of immediate concern to physicians trying to treat the acute episodes was the real nature of the inciting event and what could be done about it. The history of myocardial infarction and the role of thrombosis in its genesis was a tortuous one and, in terms of the totality of medical history, a relatively recent one.

The modern history of coronary heart disease can be dated to William Heberden's presentation of "a disease of the breast" before the Royal College of Physicians of London in 1768, and published four years later in 1772.[1] In his description of patients with "angina" (chest discomfort usually on exertion), the cardiac cause of which he did not refer to, he stated that "there are long intervals of perfect health" which might well have corresponded to asymptomatic or relatively asymptomatic periods between an initial non-fatal myocardial infarction and any subsequent episodes. Nonetheless, for a period of over 125 years the belief took hold that all anginal patients died suddenly and unexpectedly.

In 1880 another landmark publication was Carl Weigert's report on the pathology among such patients, indicating the causal connection between coronary thrombosis (blood clot) or atherosclerosis (fat depositions in the walls of the vessels) and myocardial infarction.[2] It would be many years, however, before the level of sophistication in chemistry, pharmacology and other scientific disciplines would be elevated to a point at which such knowledge could be applied to the treatment and prevention of coronary heart disease.

Then, around the turn of the nineteenth into the twentieth century, revelations about possible survival following acute myocardial infarction eventually revolutionized the clinical approach to the disease. A milestone was the report of George Dock, which he presented before the Alumni Association of the Medical Department of the University of Buffalo in 1896.[3] In his discussion of four coronary patients he included the discussion of one who survived for a week following the onset of the attack. In 1910 two Russian investigators , Obrastzow and Straschesko, presented two additional cases of acute myocardial infarction diagnosed clinically before death ensued.[4] Best known among such reports are those of Chicago physician James B. Herrick, who first suggested in 1910 that belief in the universal sudden death terminating coronary heart disease might be erroncous.[5] His better known 1912 article presented clinical descriptions of patients with acute myocardial infarction without sudden death, including one autopsy result.[6] In it he credited Dock and the Russians with having drawn similar conclusions previously. Although these views were not adopted quickly, they gradually took hold among the profession, aided by the appearance of electrocardiographic criteria for the process that appeared a few years later.[7] Now that it was realized that many patients did not die suddenly before anything could be done about it, the possibility arose that treatment of the acute event could be instituted in such patients. To decide upon the proper treatment however, physicians would have to be knowledgeable about the precise nature of the cause.

There have been a number of excellent reviews on the history of coronary heart disease.[8] Here I would like to focus on just three aspects of the subject. First, the historical basis upon which coronary thrombosis became associated with acute myocardial infarction; second, the developments that led to the questioning of this relationship and the opposing camps that arose; and finally, a recounting of the research that led to the resolution of this dispute and the lessons it teaches us.

The historical basis for relating coronary thrombosis to acute myocardial infarction.

Early accounts of post-mortem findings in patients who had died from coronary heart disease uniformly noted hardening or "ossification" of the coronary vessels. Following these were descriptions of autopsy findings in which thrombi were found within the coronary arteries. Almost without exception, these articles were in the form of anecdotal reports. Perhaps the earliest was that of Vulpian in 1866.[9] In a 75 year-old woman with a previous stroke and who died from a ruptured ventricular aneurysm (a bulging due to weakness in the muscle wall) he found an old blood clot in a coronary artery. In 1872 Quain reported the plugging of a coronary artery by a clot at the autopsy of one of his patients who had suffered anginal pains prior to death.[10] In the same year Rindfleisch, in his manual of pathology, clearly distinguished among different types of cardiac atrophy. Regarding the type related to coronary heart disease he stated, "Atheromatous degeneration of the coronary arteries with plugging of their larger branches by thrombus may be regarded in every instance as the cause of this dangerous lesion."[11] No numbers, however, were provided.

Other individual case reports appeared. Armand Hammer in 1878 is generally credited as the first physician to recognize the symptoms of coronary occlusion pre-mortem in a patient.[12] It is clear, however, that this was not a case of coronary thrombosis arising *in situ,* but most likely a case of infective endocarditis of the aortic valve with the vegetation (a collection of bacteria and reactive inflammatory material) extending into a coronary orifice. Leyden, commenting on the various clinical patterns of coronary heart disease in 1883, included a total of nine autopsies in his report.[13] Among these, only two showed coronary thrombi, one of which was suspected to have been embolic in nature. Ludvig Hektoen was ahead of his time in suspecting that coronary heart disease was not always a case of sudden precipitous death. However, the only autopsied case of coronary occlusion he reported (1892) was embolic in nature (i.e. the occluding thrombus arose elsewhere in the circulatory system and traveled to the heart, finally lodging in a coronary artery).[14]

George Dock's fourth patient, the one shown to have survived for a week following the onset of his myocardial infarction, is the one most referred to and who proved to have a "red thrombus" in the left coronary artery at autopsy. What of the other three patients? One was obviously syphilitic, and the ostial occlusion of one coronary artery could well have been related to this disease. In the other two patients, who both died suddenly, there was a coronary atheroma described in one and a thrombus superimposed upon an atheromatous coronary artery in the other. Herrick would eventually report on his experience with 200 patients with coronary heart disease.[15] However, among all of these, only three autopsies were performed, all showing coronary thrombosis.

What was the opinion on all this of Sir William Osler, the greatest physician of his time? He gave his valedictory on the subject of angina pectoris as a Lumleian Lecture before the Royal College of Physicians of London in 1910. Later observers have noted that Osler played down the importance of coronary disease as a clinical entity early in his career, and that for most of his professional life he saw only a few hospital cases with angina pectoris. Given his superb clinical abilities, it is unlikely that he missed diagnosing such cases, and the disease really was not as prominent as it later became. However, between the years of 1897 and 1910, the time of his Lumleian Lecture, he noted a rise in the number of cases coming to him, 208 over this period of time, Among these he autopsied 17 cases as clear-cut examples of the disease. In 13 of these he described definite severe narrowing of the coronary arteries but gave no exact numbers of coronary thromboses, stating only that

"…blocking of a branch with a fresh thrombus is very common in cases of sudden death in angina."[17]

Nearly twenty years later, belief in the thrombotic nature of coronary artery disease was still firmly entrenched despite the inconsistency of post-mortem findings.

For example, the American investigator J.T. Wearn in 1923 reported coronary thrombi in 18 of 19 patients autopsied (95 percent).[18] In contrast to this Parkinson and Bedford, British researchers working in London, reporting on 83 post-mortem examinations, found coronary thrombi in only 57 percent of recent infarctions and 36 percent of old infarctions.[19] In his monograph on the subject, tellingly entitled "Coronary Artery Thrombosis and Its Various Clinical Features," the Boston cardiologist Samuel Levine summarized his experience with 145 cases.[20] In association with his clinical observations, he reported the results of 45 autopsies. Among them a point of thrombotic occlusion of a coronary artery was found in only 23 patients. The fact that in only about half of the autopsied cases a coronary thrombus could be identified did not deter Levine or his contemporaries from holding fast to the conventional belief about coronary thrombosis and acute myocardial infarction. For decades thereafter, the terms were used almost interchangeably among doctors discussing the disease.

The somewhat spare evidentiary scaffolding of such beliefs – at least by current standards of research – would soon be shaken by newer trends in cardiovascular research and more systematic studies of large numbers of coronary patients by cardiologists and pathologists.

The rising challenge to the belief in coronary thrombosis as the cause of myocardial infarction.

By the time of the late 1930s and into the early 40s, some revision of thought about the role of coronary thrombosis in acute myocardial infarction began to take place. Perhaps a signal event in this development was the publication of a paper by Friedberg and Horn at Mount Sinai Hospital in New York City describing the absence of coronary occlusion in as many as 31 percent of their cases of fatal myocardial infarction.[21] They pointed out that this was not a new observation, citing a number of previous reports on this. This time around, however, the medical community seemed more prepared to accept such findings. Perhaps the greatest effect of this paper was to separate once and for all coronary thrombosis and myocardial infarction as pathological entities.

Important support for this view came later from another center: Boston, Massachusetts. In 1881 Julius Cohnheim had declared that the coronaries were "end arteries" after demonstrating that their ligation in dogs resulted in rapid death.[22] It became the accepted view that in man, following acute coronary artery occlusion, death would also quickly ensue because of the absence of coronary collaterals, additional arterial branches that might supply the myocardium at risk and alter the outcome of such an event. Despite Cohnheim there were some quarters in which it was believed that, with gradually developing occlusion rather than sudden coronary occlusion, the formation of collaterals to the area at risk might take place. This belief was confirmed by post-mortem injection studies coming out of Beth Israel Hospital in Boston in 1940 and conducted by Herrman Blumgart and Monroe Schlesinger.[23] A subsequent report in 1941 supplemented these findings.[24] The studies concluded that not only could myocardial infarctions occur without coronary occlusions, but coronary occlusions could occur without myocardial infarctions resulting, provided that preceding total occlusion, gradual narrowing over time due to atherosclerosis provided an adequate stimulus for the formation of protective collaterals to the myocardium at risk.

Predictably, in response to the report of Friedberg and Horn, a number of investigative groups over subsequent years conducted their own studies concerning the roles of atherosclerosis and coronary thrombosis in myocardial infarction. At issue was not either one or the other – all agreed that thrombi could form only on diseased coronary vessels. The critical question was whether atherosclerosis alone was the culprit or whether superimposed coronary thrombi upon previously diseased coronaries precipitated acute myocardial infarction. The numbers of autopsies performed among these newer studies were often larger than in the earlier reports, and serial section of the coronaries with microscopic examination was included to detect thrombotic occlusions that might have been missed on simple gross inspection by the naked eye. A sampling, in chronological order, of some of the more prominent of these is shown in Table 4.1.[25] Note the diversity of findings. Although the later studies indicated a higher percentage of thromboses found, the number of studies performed almost contemporaneously by equally respected and competent researchers and showing much lower percentages of coronary thrombi in acute myocardial infarction was disturbing. Also of import among some of these researchers was the belief that coronary thrombosis might have occurred as the result of the myocardial infarction and not the other way around.[26]

Table 4.1. Coronary Thrombosis in Acute Myocardial Infarction

Year	Authors	# Patients	Thrombi Found (%)
1941	Miller et al.	143	66
1956	Branwood et al.	61	21
1960	Spain et al.	265	50
1964	Ehrlich et al.	38	50
1972	Roberts et al.	107	39
1972	Sinapius	206	97
1976	Davis et al.	500	95

What were some of the factors that might have caused the under-reporting of coronary thrombosis in some of these studies? 1) Studies that included patients dying within an hour of symptoms must surely have included those with significant coronary narrowing precipitating fatal arrhythmias in the absence of an occluding thrombus. 2) Inadequate serial sectioning of the coronaries, usually performed at 3 mm to 5 mm intervals along the arteries may have missed some ultra-short occluding coronary thrombi of only a millimeter in length. 3) There was often difficulty in distinguishing older organized thrombi from other types of pathology in diseased arteries. 4) The use of different criteria of what constituted an acute myocardial infarction pathologically resulted in the inclusion of some patients with minor myocardial or endocardial (inner wall) scarring that did not represent infarctions. 5) Some investigators excluded "non-obstructive" thrombi, not realizing that these may have represented occluding thrombi that had been partially dissolved by intrinsic fibrinolytic mechanisms as had been demonstrated in human pulmonary thrombi.[27] Experimentally, at least, the same phenomenon was found in dogs in whom coronary thrombi had been produced.[28] But until irrefutable new evidence for coronary thrombosis would appear, such explanations would be resisted in many quarters.

The introduction of selective coronary arteriography by Mason Sones in 1962 was a major step forward in delineating the status of the coronary arteries in humans *in vivo*.[29]

This procedure, in which radiopaque dye was injected into coronary arteries and their structure visualized with X-ray, may have led physicians to de-emphasize the role of coronary thrombosis in acute myocardial infarction. One pattern of coronary atherosclerosis involves the gradual progression of coronary lumen narrowing until such a point at which normal resting coronary flow can exist, but with exercise the increased need for coronary blood flow cannot be met. Typical angina on effort is the clinical manifestation of this, and it was these patients that presented for cardiac catheterization in whom coronary bypass surgery often yielded dramatic relief.[30] Another type of atheroma formation involves the "vulnerable plaque." These lesions often appear less severe on angiography than those described above, but are more prone to rupture due to their thin fibrous caps separating their contents from the coronary artery lumen. Once the cap separates, the contents of the atheroma, mixing with the blood within the artery, leads to platelet aggregation and other clotting mechanisms to produce the occluding thrombus with a resultant myocardial infarction.[31] The association of the vulnerable plaque with producing coronary thrombi would only become apparent more than a decade after the introduction of coronary arteriography, when it was learned that such studies could be performed in acute myocardial infarction in patients with relative safety. Finally, growing awareness of the importance of diet and the role of blood cholesterol levels, as important as this was in the genesis of coronary artery disease, tended to downplay any associated role of thrombosis in causing acute myocardial infarction.

Initial efforts to apply anticoagulant therapy early in the treatment of acute myocardial infarction and then long-term did not serve to further the cause of the coronary thrombosis hypothesis. In addition to some flaws in study design (e.g. failure to achieve true randomization in the selection of treatment and control groups), trials of anticoagulation for acute myocardial infarction were not very encouraging; any improvement in survival statistics were more likely due to prevention of thromboembolic complications (e.g. fatal pulmonary embolism) than in the treatment of the offending coronary artery thrombus itself; and the risk of bleeding, sometimes life-threatening, was another consideration.[32] In retrospect, such findings could have been expected. The early agents used for anticoagulation , coumadin derivatives, and later heparin, while preventing clot formation, have no effect of dissolving thrombi once formed. However, long-term studies using these agents following an initial myocardial infarction were similarly disappointing in preventing recurrences.[33]

A particularly vexing aspect of pathological studies involving acute myocardial infarction were some that emphasized the presence of intramural coronary artery hemorrhages, those within the wall of the coronary artery, and not in contact with the lumen, in most cases of acute infarction.[34] This suggested that the expansion of these hematomas is what caused the occlusion of the artery. If such were the case, the use of anticoagulation might not only be unhelpful, but actually contraindicated. Later studies, however, repudiated this view.[35] More recent research has indicated that such hemorrhages are incorporated into the atheromatous plaque rather than expanding into the lumen of the vessel.[36]

In 1973, at the National Heart and Lung Institute of the National Institutes of Health in Bethesda, Maryland, a workshop was convened in which the various investigators who had grappled with the problem discussed their views.[37] Attempts were made to reconcile the discordant findings among different groups of investigators, noting the integral relations between the alterations in the arterial wall (i.e. atheroma) and thromboses that had been reported in the past. However, the end result, for the most part, consisted of a restatement of positions previously held. Although the joint conclusion emphasized the importance of coronary thrombosis, it also concluded that the idea that coronary thrombosis was a secondary event, following the infarction, was provocative and deserved serious consideration. So how did medical researchers find their way out of this confusing thicket of contradictory findings? What finally went right?

Establishing the role of coronary thrombosis in acute myocardial infarction.

In 1971 Marcus DeWood and his colleagues began a landmark study that, once and for all, would resolve the question of the role of coronary thrombosis in acute myocardial infarction.[38] Daring for its time, the study was performed in patients early in the course of acute myocardial infarctions. Eventually it involved 322 patients, all studied by coronary arteriography. It was completed seven years later in 1978. In patients studied within 4 hours of the event's onset, 85 percent demonstrated an occluding coronary artery thrombus on angiography. Among those studied 12 to 24 hours after the onset of symptoms, there was a decline in the frequency of thrombi, 65 percent, evidence that soon after formation coronary thrombi begin to undergo lysis. This supported the contention that among those post-mortem studies previously performed in patients who died several days after their infarction, thrombi would be reduced in size ("non-occluding") or absent. Of 79 patients rushed to surgery for coronary bypass surgery, thrombi could be extracted by Fogarty catheter from the coronaries in 85 percent. Without doubt, the predominant role of coronary thrombosis was established. This provided firm support for the report a year earlier by Rentrop on the efficacy of an intracoronary infusion of streptokinase in recanalizing acutely occluded coronary arteries in myocardial infarction.[39] Later studies, using angioscopy in patients with acute myocardial infarctions, confirmed and extended these results.[40] Later developments in imaging techniques such as computed tomography and magnetic resonance imaging provided further insights into the formation and dissolution of coronary thrombi.[41]

In the small number of infarction patients in whom coronary thrombi cannot be found, other mechanisms inducing ischemia were uncovered. Prolonged spasm of one or more coronary branches can result in sufficient impairment to blood flow so as to result in myocardial infarction. In some patients who have bands of myocardium ("bridges") running superficially across one of their coronary arteries, contraction of such muscular bands can squeeze the coronary shut sufficiently to result in coronary occlusion without thrombosis. Finally, other diseases may, secondarily, result in coronary occlusion without thrombosis (e.g. proximally dissecting aortic aneurysms, embolism of endocarditic vegetations in a coronary orifice etc.).

With the importance of coronary thrombosis in the pathogenesis of acute myocardial infarction now established, modern therapy for coronary thrombosis includes drugs that reduce platelet adhesiveness, interfere with the formation or propagation of thrombi by blocking one or more of the coagulation pathways, or actually dissolve thrombi that have already been formed.

Conclusions

There are several lessons to be learned from the coronary thrombosis controversy. A hypothesis, even when supported by insufficient or flawed evidence, may eventually turn out to be valid. The cause of many diseases may be multiple. In the controversy reviewed here, oftentimes researchers tended to champion either coronary thrombosis or atheromatous disease of the coronary arteries. Both are ultimately involved in acute myocardial infarction , with the disruption of the fibrous cap of a vulnerable plaque being the critical element in leading to coronary thrombosis. A new technique of investigation may suddenly shed light on a problem unresolved by pre-existing methods of examination. In this case, coronary arteriography and later angioscopy in living patients with acute infarctions overcame the distortions of pathological fixing and sectioning of post-mortem specimens. The long and involved investigative experience with coronary thrombosis provides an object lesson that may apply to a number of other unresolved medical mysteries that continue to plague both physicians and their patients.

REFERENCES

1. Heberden, W. Some account of a disorder of the breast. *Med Trans Coll Physns London 1772;2:59-67.*

2. Weigert C. Ueber die pathologüsche Gerinnugs-Vorgänge. *Arch Path Anat Virchow* 1880;79:87-123.

3. Dock, G. *Notes on the Coronary Arteries.* Ann Arbor, Mich.: Inland Press, 1896.

4. Obrastzow WP, Straschesko ND. Zur Kennis der Thrombose der Koronararterien des Herzens. *Zeitschr für Klin Med* 1910;71:116-132.

5. Herrick, JB. Certain popular but erroneous notions concerning angina pectoris. *J Am Med Assoc* 1910;55:1424-27.

6. Herrick, JB. Clinical features of sudden obstruction of the coronary arteries. *J Am Med Assoc* 1912;59:2015-20.

7. Pardee, HEB. An electrocardiographic sign of coronary artery obstruction. *Arch Int Med* 1920;26:244-57.

8. See Leibowitz, JO. *The History of Coronary Heart Disease.* Berkeley:University of California Press, 1970; Fye, WB. Acute myocardial infarction. A historical summary. In *Acute Myocardial Infarction,* Ed. Gersh BJ, Rahimtoola S. New York:Elsevier, 1990. p1-13; and Acierno LJ. *The History of Cardiology.* London:Parthenon, 1994.

9. Vulpian EFA. Ramollissement cerebral ancien… infarctus de la paroi du ventricule gauche du coeur coincident avec l'existence d'un caillot ancien dans l'une artères coronaries… *L'Union Medicale* 1866;29:417-419.

10. Quain R. Dilatation of the arch of the aorta and plugging and obliteration of the left coronary artery. *Trans Path Soc London* 1882;23:57-59.

11. Rindfleisch E. *Manual of Pathological Histology to Serve as an Introduction to the Study of Morbid Anatomy.* Trans. Baxter EB London:New Sydenham Soc., 1872.

12. Hammer A. A case of thrombotic occlusion of one of the coronary arteries of the heart. *Wien Med Wochnschr* 1878;28:102 (Translation in *Classic Descriptions of Disease,* Ed. Major RH. Springfield, IL:Charles C. Thomas, 1965. pp426-428.

13. Leyden E. Ueber die Sclerose der Coronar-Arterien und die davon abhängigen Krankheitszustände. *Klin Med* 1883;1:459-86.

14. Hektoen L. Embolism of the left coronary artery: sudden death. *Med News* 1892;61:210-21.

15. Herrick JB, Nuzum FR. Angina pectoris. Clinical experience with two hundred cases. *J Am Med Assoc* 1918;70:67-70.

16. Herrick JB. Thrombosis of the coronary arteries. *J Am Med Assoc* 1919;72:387-90.

17. Osler W. Angina pectoris. *The Lancet* 1910;1:697-702, 839-44, p.840.

18. Wearn JT. Thrombosis of the coronary arteries with infarction of the heart. *Am J Med Sci* 1923;165:250-76.

19. Parkinson J, Bedford DE. Cardiac infarction and coronary thrombosis. *The Lancet* 1928;1:4-11.

20. Levine SA. *Coronary Thrombosis and Its Various Clinical Features.* Baltimore:Williams and Wilkins, 1929.

21. Friedberg CK, Horn H. Acute myocardial infarction not due to coronary occlusion. *J Am Med Assoc* 1939;112:1675-79.

22. Cohnheim J, v. Schultess-Rechberg A. Ueber die Folgen der Kranzarterienversüchliessung für das Herz. *Virchows Arch Path Anat* 1881;85:503-7.

23. Blumgart HL, Schlesinger MJ, Davis D. Studies on the relation of the clinical manifestations of angina pectoris, coronary thrombosis and myocardial infarction to the pathologic findings. With particular reference to the collateral circulation. *Am Heart J* 1940;19:1-91.

24. Blumgart HL, Schlesinger MJ, Zoll PM. Angina pectoris, coronary failure and acute myocardial infarction. The role of coronary occlusions and collateral circulation. *J Am Med Assoc* 1941;116:91-97.

25. Miller DR, Burchell HB, Edwards J. Myocardial infarction with and without occlusion. *Arch Int Med* 1951;88:597-604; Branwood AW, Montgomery GL. Observations of the morbid anatomy of coronary artery disease. *Scot Med J* 1956;1:367-75; Spain DM, Brandess VA. The relationship of coronary thrombosis to coronary atherosclerosis and ischemic heart

disease. A necropsy study covering a period of 25 years. *Am J Med Sci* 1960;240:701-10; Ehrlich JC, Shinohara Y. Low incidence of coronary thrombosis in myocardial infarction. *Arch Path* 1964;78:432-45; Roberts WC, Macmillan B. The frequency and significance of coronary arterial thrombi and other observations in fatal acute myocardial infarction. A study of 107 necropsy hearts. *Am J Med* 1972;52:425-43; Sinapius D. Beziehungen zwischen Koronarthrombosen und Myokardinfarkten. *Dtch Med Wochenschr* 1972;97:443-48; Davies MJ, Woolf N, Robertson WB. Pathology of acute myocardial infarction with particular reference to occlusive coronary thrombi. *Brit Heart J* 1976;38:659-64.

26. See note 25, Branwood, Observations on Morbid Anatomy; Ehrlich, Low incidence of coronary thrombosis; and Roberts, Frequency of thrombi.

27. Fred HL, Axelrod A, Lewis JM, Alexander JK. Rapid dissolution of pulmonary thromboembolism in man. *J Am Med Assoc* 1966;196:1137-39.

28. Weisse AB, Lehan PH, Ettinger PO, Moschos CB, Regan TJ. The fate of experimentally produced coronary artery thrombosis. *Am J Cardiol* 1969;23:229-37.

29. Sones FM, Shirey EK. Cine Coronary Arteriography. *Mod Concepts Cardiovasc Dis* 1962;31:735-38.

30. See Favoloro RG in Weisse AB. *Heart to Heart. The Twentieth Century Battle Against Cardiac Disease. An Oral History.* New Brunswick, NJ: Rutgers Univ. Press, 2002.

31. Fuster V, Badimon L, Badimon JJ, Cheseboro JH. The pathogenesis of coronary artery disease and the acute coronary syndromes. *New Engl J Med* 1992;326:242-50, 310-18.

32. Wright IS, Marple CD, Beck DF. Report of the Committee for Evaluation of Anticoagulants in the Treatment of Coronary Thrombosis and Myocardial Infarction. *Am Heart J* 1948;36:801-15; Report of the Working Party on Anticoagulant Therapy in Coronary Thrombosis to the Medical Research Council. Assessment of short-term anticoagulant administration after cardiac infarction. *Brit Med J* 1969;1:335-42; Anticoagulants in myocardial infarction. Results of a cooperative clinical trial. *J Am Med Assoc* 1973;225:724-29.

33. Long-term anticoagulation after myocardial infarction: Final report of the Veterans Administration Cooperative Study. *J Am Med Assoc* 1969;297:2263-67; Meuwissen OGAT, Vervoorn AC, Cohn C, et al. Double-blind trial of long-term anticoagulant treatment after myocardial infarction. *Acta Med Scand* 1969;186:361-68; Collaborative analysis of long-term anticoagulant administration following acute myocardial infarction. An international anticoagulant review group. *Lancet* 1970;1:203-09

34. This was based primarily on the report of J.C. Paterson: Vascularization and hemorrhage of the intima of atherosclerotic coronary arteries. *Arch Path* 1936;22:313-24. Supporting and extending these findings were: Wartman WB. Occlusion of the coronary arteries by hemorrhage into their walls. *Am Heart J* 1938;15:458-70; and Horn H, Finkelstein L. Atherosclerosis of the coronary arteries and the mechanism of their occlusion. *Am Heart J* 1940;19:655-82.

35. This is summarized in Crawford T. Morphological aspects in the pathogenesis of atherosclerosis. *J Atheroscl Res* 1961;1:3-25. See also Friedman M, van den Bovencamp GJ. The pathogenesis of a coronary thrombus. *Am J Path* 1966;48:19-44; and Friedman M. *Pathogenesis of Coronary Artery Disease.* New York:McGraw Hill, 1969.

36. Kolodgie FD, Gold HK, Burke AP et al. Intraplaque hemorrhage and progression of coronary atheroma. *New Engl J Med* 2003;349:2316-25.

37. Chandler AB, Chapman I, Erhardt LR et al. Coronary thrombosis in myocardial infarction. Report of a workshop on the role of coronary thrombosis in the pathogenesis of acute myocardial infarction. *Am J Cardiol* 1974;34:823-33.

38. DeWood MA, Spores J, Notske R et al. Prevalence of total coronary occlusion during the early hours of transmural myocardial infarction. *New Engl J Med* 1980;303:897-902.

39. Rentrop KP, Blanke H, Karsch R et al. Acute myocardial infarction: Intracoronary application of nitroglycerine and streptokinase. *Clin Cardiol* 1979;2:354-63.

40. Forrester JS, Litvack F, Grundfest W, Hickey A, A perspective of coronary disease as seen through the arteries of living man.

Circulation 1987;75:505-13; Mizuno K, Myamoto A, Satomura K et al. Angioscopic coronary macromorphology in patients with acute coronary syndromes. *The Lancet* 1991;337:809-12; Mizuno K, Satomura K, Myamoto A et al. Angioscopic evaluation of coronary artery thrombi in acute coronary syndromes. *New Engl J Med* 1992;326:287-91.

41. Sanz J, Poon M. Evaluation of ischemic heart disease with magnetic resonance and computed tomography. *Expert Rev Cardiovasc Ther* 2004;2:601-15.

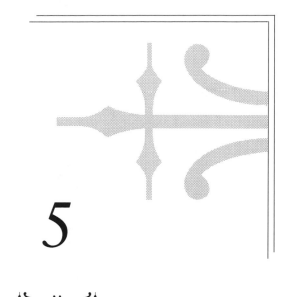

5

CONFESSIONS OF CREEPING OBSOLESCENCE

THE MEMORY OF JAMES B. Herrick (1861-1954) is revered by hematologists and cardiologists alike. He was considered to be one of their own by both groups of specialists. In 1910, it was Herrick who first described those peculiarly shaped red blood corpuscles characteristic of sickle cell anemia.[1] Two years later, in another landmark paper, he pointed out that sudden obstruction of a coronary artery did not always result in immediate death.[2] Herrick acknowledged that he was not the first to recognize the clinical features of what we now call acute myocardial infarction and, indeed, quoted the writings of others to support his own arguments about the nonlethal coronary occlusions. However, Herrick's report undoubtedly had the most influence in spreading the word and leading future physicians toward better recognition, treatment and prevention of coronary heart disease.

Given the period during which Herrick reached his medical maturity, it is highly unlikely that he ever considered himself exclusively a hematologist or cardiologist. Even to have called him an internist would have been premature. "Internists" got their start in Germany during the early 1880s, but the designation arrived here a good deal later. It was not until 1945 that the American Medical Association actually replaced "the practice of medicine" with "internal medicine."[3]

Although he founded the Society of Internal Medicine of Chicago in 1915, Herrick, in his prime, would have most likely been simply called a physician (or possibly a consultant) with a particular interest in matters involving the cardiovascular or hematological systems. Whatever one calls him, Herrick, for all his accomplishments and success, was prey to the lifelong affliction of all internists: the difficulty of keeping up with such a massive and all-encompassing field. So concerned was he about his ignorance of chemistry, which was coming to dominate medical thought and research at the beginning of the 20th century, that he temporarily abandoned a busy private practice in 1904 at the age of forty-three in order to update his knowledge. The process included a trip to Germany for further training in this discipline.

Even the patron saint of internal medicine, Sir William Osler, was not immune to pangs of inadequacy. In his memoirs, Herrick recalls a meeting with Osler at an American Medical Association convention in 1902 when, confronted with an array of biochemical representations placed on the blackboard by one speaker, Osler expressed the longing to be nineteen again and able to "do it all over."[4] Whatever his misgivings about the state of his knowledge, Osler had not been deterred from writing a textbook of medicine a decade earlier – and a darned good one at that. Given the continued expansion of our specialty, who among us would have the temerity to attempt a similar feat today? Who would even attempt a monograph on a subspecialty without the assistance of super specialists within the field?

As a cardiologist, I have always liked to think of myself as an internist first. As such, I have accepted the chronic anxiety about keeping up that comes with the territory, but it has not been easy. The seeds of my own self-doubt were already sown by the time I had left medical school. Sir Hans A. Krebs was primarily responsible.

Practically our entire course in biochemistry was devoted to the elucidation of the citric acid cycle, for which Krebs, incidentally, with Fritz A. Lipmann was awarded a Nobel Prize in Medicine in 1953. At each lecture our professor would chalk up another segment of the saga until at the final session, the whole thing appeared on blackboards lining the large lecture hall, and our professor, unwittingly in deference to Kreb's Teutonic origins, had drawn all the leitmotifs together in a Gotterdammerung-like exposition.

In fifty years of medical practice, I have yet to bring the Krebs cycle to the bedside, for all its importance and brilliance.

It was not only biochemistry that seared my soul. Take hematology as another example of my growing ineptitude. Somewhere back in the dim, distant past, the clotting scheme was as delightfully comprehensible as it was incomplete. Prothrombin-to-thrombin-to fibrin had a Tinker-to-Evers-to-Chance simplicity that was 100 percent American in some way. But even when I was a medical student in the late 1950s, those Roman numbered clotting factors were beginning to clutter up the picture: Factors V, VII, IX and X were almost familiar to me by the time I graduated in 1958. But new ones kept coming. And to further complicate the picture, for every new clotting factor there seemed to be an associated anticlotting factor on the horizon. "Cascade" is the name they now give to the clotting process, and I have nightmarish visions of factor MDCCXVII and all its predecessors engulfing me in a monstrous lava-like flow of hemic ooze. All this without even getting into the tissue factors involved in the process.

The varieties of white blood cells also seem to be expanding exponentially. It is no longer adequate to define them on the basis of their morphology or staining properties. Each new type is now categorized on the basis of its performance. It is either a killer cell or a helper cell or some other type of well-adjusted or malevolent character.

It is just as bad with prostaglandins. Ever since Ulf von Euler got the ball rolling in the 1930s, they seem to have appeared in almost every organ system. But in medical practice they remain at a distance, like some highly respected foreign guests with whom, because of the language barrier, we cannot adequately communicate.

Henderson-Hasselbalch is to acid-base chemistry what wheat is to bread, but my only contribution in practice was to primly correct medical students who, inadvertently, omitted pronouncing the second "l" in Hasselbalch. It is true that I now find the "anion gap" not totally confusing and am even able to calculate it on occasion despite the persistent gaps, I am sure, in my understanding.

Nobel laureate Arthur Kornberg once sent me a reprint of his paper entitled, "For the Love of Enzymes." He even used this title for his autobiography.[5] Loving enzymes was a bit much for me, but I have tried my level best to at least like them. Unfortunately, I must confess, they simply don't seem to like me.

Infectious disease is another source of dismay for the internist who would like to keep abreast of recent developments. Long ago, however, I gave up on this as well. As a self-respecting clinical cardiologist and busy echocardiographer, I took second place to no one in my ability to diagnose infective endocarditis (a heart valve infection). But once the diagnosis was made, I despaired of ever choosing the right antibiotic or combination of the day or week, and turned that decision over to the "ID boys." There was too much danger of selecting a third generation cephalosporin when only a fourth would do – unless we were already on to the fifth or sixth.

And so it goes through the vast realm we call internal medicine: gastroenterology, immunology, endocrinology, rheumatology and the rest. This did not mean that, as a cardiologist I did not have my own areas of esoterica with which to confuse other internists. In the past cardiologists could dazzle by judging among several different kinds of digitalis preparations. Then we developed our classification of anti-arrhythmics. Later came an array of beta blockers, calcium channel blockers and ACE inhibitors about which we could demonstrate our superior knowledge. But this only serves to emphasize the hopelessness of effort in the entire body of practicing internists.

And yet, quixotically, I persist. I once counted the number of journals I read or scanned. An incomplete list included five general medical journals, four internal medicine journals, ten cardiovascular disease journals, two basic science journals covering cardiovascular physiology and three scientific journals with broader scope, not to mention the New York Times. I am not sure how much they helped me keep up to date.

The late Sir George Pickering, Regius Professor of Medicine at Oxford, was noted for his research on hypertension, but he was no slouch on problems concerned with learning the new medicine and doing away with the old. He also had a devilishly witty way of putting things. In a slim volume containing his views on medical education, he dispensed with the old fogies of medicine as follows: "Where there is death there is hope."[6]

As the intellectual deadwood within the medical community gets removed, our students, who did their medical teething on rings of recombinant DNA, will undoubtedly be less confused by what is new in medicine, and this, I suppose is how progress is made. In the meantime the rest of us must continue to live with our doubts about our ability to fulfill our early hopes and expectations.

But there is some solace to be found in this dilemma. It is just such insecurity about the extent of our knowledge that spurs us on to continued self-education. Because of our concern about being able to do right by our patients, we try that much harder – and perhaps the care we provide might be just a little bit better.

REFERENCES

1. Herrick JB. Peculiar elongated and sickle-shaped red blood corpuscles in a case of severe anemia. *Trans Assoc Am Phys* 1910;25:553.

2.   Herrick JB. Clinical features of sudden obstruction of the coronary arteries. *J Am Med Assoc* 1912;59:2015.

3. Bean WB. Origin of the term "internal medicine." *New Engl J Med* 1982;306:182

4. Herrick JB. *Memories of Eighty Years.* Chicago: Univ. of Chicago Press, 1949

5. Kornberg A. *For the Love of Enzymes.* Boston: Harvard Univ. Press, 1989.

6. Pickering G. *Quest for Excellence in Medical Education.* Oxford: Oxford Univ. Press, 1978, p44.

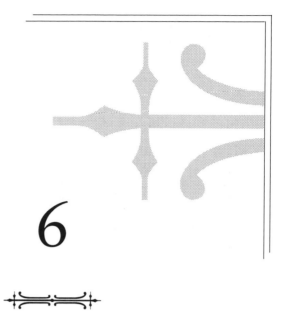

6

ON FIRST LOOKING INTO JARCHO'S LEIBOWITZ: THE CLINICIAN AS MEDICAL HISTORIAN

Not LONG AGO, IN the course of doing some research that centered upon the role of coronary thrombosis in acute myocardial infarction, I learned of a monograph on the history of coronary disease that was considered a standard source on the subject and thought this might be helpful. It was written by Joshua Leibowitz, a professor at the Hadassah medical school in Jerusalem.[1] I obtained a used copy through an Internet book dealer. When I opened to the first page I was amazed to see the beginning of a detailed analysis by none other than Saul Jarcho (Figure 6.1), who was using this as his review copy for the *Bulletin of the The History of Medicine* over 30 years ago.[2] Not only were his notes exhaustive but one I found, commenting on a source in Hebrew, was actually written in Hebrew.

The name Saul Jarcho was not unknown to me. As a budding cardiologist in the 1960s I began my subscription to the American Journal of Cardiology and noted frequent contributions by Jarcho –

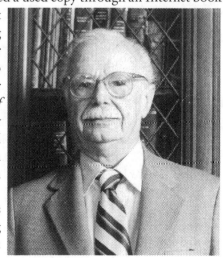

Figure 6.1 Saul Jarcho (1906-2000). Courtesy of the New York Academy of Medicine Library

not a cardiologist, incidentally – on the history of cardiovascular medicine. Amazingly, between 1958 and 1976 he published more than 100 annotated extracts from the older literature on cardiovascular disease and they were remarkably well informed. This was only one aspect of Jarcho's extensive medical historical research. My delight at rediscovering Jarcho was not unlike that expressed in sonnet form by Keats: On First Looking Into Chapman's Homer.

This new encounter with Jarcho so many years later stimulated my curiosity about him. I found a special section of the *Journal of Urban Health/ Bulletin of the New York Academy of Medicine* that constituted a tribute to Jarcho and included a short autobiographical essay.[3] It was from this and comments of others contributing to this special issue that I learned a good deal about this unusual man.

Saul Jarcho was born in New York City in 1906 to a family that had emigrated from the Ukraine in the late 19th century. His father, who had received some medical training in Russia prior to arriving in the United States, completed his medical studies at Columbia University's College of Physicians and Surgeons.

Saul was something of a *wunderkind*. He was admitted to Harvard College as a pre-medical student at the age of 15 but his father had him wait a year because of his tender age. Before matriculating, Saul, on attending a reception by President Lowell of Harvard, was advised by him: "Were I you and intending to enter medicine I should concentrate on anything but chemistry and zoology." Jarcho immediately discarded his plans for a program heavily steeped in the sciences and majored in English Literature. He made good on the scientific courses missed in Cambridge during summers at Columbia College in New York City. Although he was immersed in English Literature at Harvard there was a standard course in history that, according to Jarcho "…included everything that happened between the fall of the Roman Empire and the Wednesday before the final examination. There was not a word about the nature, purpose or value of history. *This led to an oath that I would never touch history again* [italics added]."

Nonetheless, after receiving his bachelor's degree at Harvard he spent a year at Columbia obtaining a masters degree in Roman Literature. This included a summer at the American Academy in Rome studying Latin. He then obtained a medical degree from Columbia's College of Physicians and Surgeons, with summers spent at the School of Tropical Medicine in Puerto Rico. After obtaining his M.D. degree he spent roughly three years in New York hospitals in what amounted to a rotating internship and residency. This was followed by three years in pathology at Johns Hopkins. He became board certified in Internal Medicine in 1950. For the rest of his professional life he would be based in New York at Columbia and especially Mt. Sinai Hospital where he practiced internal medicine until 1980.

This long stint in New York City was interrupted only by World War II when, between 1942 and 1946 he served in Military Intelligence in the United States Army. Throughout his career as a busy internist Jarcho maintained an active parallel one in medical history without, I pointedly add, any formal training in history. His intellect and curiosity were reflected in the wide range of his literary output with over five hundred contributions by the time of his death in 2000.

Jarcho received many awards and occupied many positions of distinction and responsibility. Yet, with all his erudition, Jarcho was frequently noted as well for his wit and humor by those who knew him. This was quite a man and he represented a very special kind of scholar, one almost absent on the current medical scene: the clinician-historian.

What especially impressed me about Jarcho was his linguistic ability. In 1940, suspecting that with Allied forces heading eventually for North Africa and having a need for M.D.s with some fluency in Arabic, he essentially learned the language on his own – adding it to his knowledge of German, French, Italian, Latin, Hebrew and – lest we forget – some Anglo-Saxon as well. It was his exposure to both the Italian language and culture in particular that I believe led to his historical research on a number of aspects of Italian medicine that would unlikely to have been addressed by others without such an intellectual foundation. Merely listing some of the titles of Jarcho's papers reveals the broad breadth and depth of his oeuvre:

- The Medical Imprints of Giambattista Bodoni
- Concept of Heart Failure from Avicenna to Albertini
- The Hunt for a Manuscript on Cinchona
- The Style of Zucutus Lusitanus and Its Origins
- Two Maps on an Early Treatise on Epidemiology
- A Note on the Autopsy of Oliver Cromwell
- Some Historical Problems with the Study of Egyptian Mummies
- Dr. Nicholas Tulp and Rembrandt's Anatomy Lesson

Although Jarcho was particularly gifted in linguistics his was not an isolated case. Many of his contemporaries, especially those in academic medicine, had at least a reading knowledge of Latin and modern foreign languages which enabled them to keep up with the medical literature of the time.

Many of our grandparents and great grandparents would have recognized a time when no person was considered properly educated without a knowledge of Greek and Latin, a centuries' old belief in what was considered proper preparation for learned individuals. In more modern times, perhaps from the seventeenth or eighteenth centuries up to the time of the Second World War when much of the advanced medical learning was still emanating from laboratories, universities and hospitals in France and Germany, lack of a reading knowledge in these languages and, to a lesser extent, Italian, was undoubtedly a distinct disadvantage.

This was certainly recognized by the faculty at the Johns Hopkins Medical School at the time of its founding. Admissions were limited to those with a reading knowledge of at least French and German. Although some students found this off-putting, the more scholarly inclined felt this to be a reflection of the institution's excellence and it was this kind of student Hopkins wanted to attract.[4]

With the deluge of new knowledge in medicine over the last century and the pre-eminence of American medicine over the last half-century or more, it is understandable why American medical schools have discontinued such requirements of their entering students. Nonetheless, the lack of such language skills cannot help but deprive any clinician/historian of a valuable asset in conducting medical historical research. Concern about this deficiency among professional historians has also been expressed. A recent publication of the American Historical Society on the education of historians for the twenty-first century notes the reduction in requirements for language proficiency within many Ph.D. programs in history where knowledge of language has become "…a hurdle rather than a resource."[5]

During my own lifetime as I approached medicine as a profession and then matured within its confines there were many physicians and other biological scientists who were prominent and influenced my views and those of my contemporaries on the place of medicine and its development within society: Lester King, Victor Robinson, Lewis Thomas, Henry Wilcox Haggard, Hans Zinsser, René Dubos and others. Finally there was Paul de Kruif, whose golly-gosh-gee-whiz style we would all consider "corny" today but whose book, *Microbe Hunters*, probably encouraged more American students to pursue a career in medicine than any other book of the time and, perhaps, any since.[6] Where are such figures today to teach and inspire newer generations of physicians about their professional heritage? It has been suggested that with the birth of the Internet they are more likely to rush to their computers than the medical library for such information. Yet, at least one inquiry into the reading habits of medical neophytes indicates that they are still turning to books; only the iconic authors of yore of been replaced by others.[7] (The enormous popularity of books like *The Da Vinci Code* and The Harry Potter phenomenon are reassuring developments indicating that the future will be filled with as many book lovers as in the past.) Another possible reason for the paucity of easily recognized clinician-historians today is that there simply are not that many around anymore; that today's clinicians have been become either disinterested in or discouraged from even entering the medical history arena.

An often-mentioned source of such prejudice might be the preeminent organization for medical history in this country, the American Association for the History of Medicine (AAHM). Most people today might not be aware of it, but as Genevieve Miller documented in her account of the first fifty years of the AAHM, it began as an exclusively M.D. affair.[8] Interestingly, she notes toward the end of her paper, "The programs include an increasing number of papers by professional historians and graduate students in social and intellectual history who are discovering fertile sources of investigation in medical history." And later on, "As the years progressed, the physician members were joined by medical librarians, professional historians and other non-medical members."[9] Ironically, thirty years later many physicians would complain that the clinicians were not simply joined by these newcomers but effectively squeezed out by them. Yet in 2002 among the over 1100 members of the AAHM physicians still constituted the largest sub-group within the membership (43 percent). However, at the 2002 annual meeting of the AAHM they represented only 19 percent of the attendees and merely 11 percent of the presenters.

In 2004 Dr. Robert D. Hudson, a distinguished senior medical historian published a paper entitled "Medical History Without Medicine" in which he lamented "…the virtual disappearance of physicians as historians of medicine," and "…their waning active involvement in medical history."[10] In reviewing the 2003 program of the AAHM annual meeting his analysis of the abstracts presented was similar to that for 2002: among 95 presenters he found that only 13 percent held M.D. degrees.

Concerned about the declining participation of clinicians at their annual meetings, the officers of the AAHM in 2005 tabulated more recent data. For the 2005 meeting they found that of the abstracts submitted only 16 percent (23/146) came from M.D.s. Whereas 65 percent of the abstracts submitted by historians were accepted for presentation, and 56 percent (5/9) of submissions from M.D./Ph.D.s were chosen for the program, only 19 percent (2/14) of those from M.D.s lacking historian credentials were selected. For whatever reasons, not only were M.D.s expressing less interest in the meeting but they also were encountering less interest from the program committees in charge.

Perhaps a truer representation of the current status of clinicians in the field of medical history can be found by examining what actually winds up in the literature as completed research. The official publication of the AAHM is the *Bulletin of the History of Medicine* (BHM). Appearing quarterly, with each issue usually featuring four or five full-length articles, it represents a major repository of English language research in the field. I took it upon myself to analyze its contents as a reflection of the current status of medical historical research.

The task was basically twofold: to determine something about the types of article that were being published and who it was that was doing the writing. To accomplish this I started with a recent issue of the journal (Winter 2005) and, working backwards, selected 100 full-length articles, excluding those that were part of symposia. As I read each article I asked myself, without casting a shadow on the authors of the many excellent papers involved, "Would a knowledge of some medical specialty (e.g. surgery, obstetrics, cardiology etc.) have been helpful for anyone addressing this topic?" Although some personal prejudices may have crept into this selection reasonable objectivity was assured by the fact that the degrees and affiliations of the authors are not listed on the title page and that I recognized the names of only seven of the 114 authors of the total 100 papers. After completing this phase of the operation I then checked for all the authors' academic credentials and academic affiliations. These I learned from the "authors' information" section at the back of each issue, the AAHM and other membership lists, the Internet and through direct contact by email. This author information was complete for all but seven individuals.

Who were the people whose work was being published? Over 80 percent were either Ph.D.s, almost all in history, or on their way to achieving this status. Sixteen percent (18/114) had degrees in medicine. All but two of the 114 had some academic affiliation, either with a university or research institute.

Among the 100 articles only 30 met my criteria for being medically oriented. For these 30 articles the author or one of the authors was an M.D. in 13 or 43 percent. The degree of clinician participation therefore turned out to be low but not quite as low as the abstract reviews had predicted. Despite some of the small numbers involved and some unavoidable element of subjectivity, any reasonable person, I believe, would still have to concede that both clinicians and the kind of material that would most engage their attention was underrepresented. One finding of interest was that five of the thirteen physicians mentioned above had obtained training in history either at the master's or doctorate level. Importantly, what could not be determined were the number of important topics of a technical nature that were not being addressed within the pages of the BHM because insufficient numbers of clinician historians with the necessary qualifications were engaging in this kind of work.

Where are we heading? In recent years in an attempt to improve patient care and insure accountability within medicine there has been an increasing tendency toward certification and recertification among the medical specialties.[11] In this age of credentialing it is not surprising that such tendencies may have infiltrated attitudes toward the practice of medical history research as well. Although no patient ever died or became permanently disabled as the result of a misspelled name, a false date or misinterpreted manuscript, it is hard to argue that such mandatory training would not raise the quality of such research performed by clinicians. Although this may be the wave of the future this would be a long-term goal. For the present, instituting such requirements now would only serve to discourage even more physicians without such training from making possibly important contributions. Indeed, there have been voices raised in dissent to such requirements even from established individuals within the professional historian community. Owsei Temkin (1902-2002) of Johns Hopkins was truly a grand old man of medical history. He was an M.D. who, incidentally, never felt the need to pursue a degree in history even though he had devoted his entire professional life to this discipline. In his last collection of essays he comments, "Competence in historical research is indispensable. But how it has been acquired is irrelevant and should not be determined by academic formality."[12] Another prominent historian, John. C. Burnham, has written, "The question was the product, whether social history or technical history or some combination."[13]

What might we conclude from all of this?

It is obvious, at least from the review of one prominent historical journal, that there is appearing in print only a small fraction of the work that could be contributed by clinicians either independently or in cooperation with professional historians. While the problem of this imbalance is serious it is by no means insoluble. It appears that a small but growing number of clinicians are seeking additional historical credentials as they enter this increasingly competitive field. Of greater importance, for the immediate future at least, is the evidence of sustained interest among a large number of clinicians in medical history by their continued membership in the AAHM. Surely more than a handful of the hundreds of physicians within the AAHM are capable of producing solid work in the field even without the benefit of formalized training in historical research methodology.

Also on the positive side of the equation is the fact that the AAHM remains a fairly open organization. Membership is still available to anyone interested and willing to pay the modest annual fee. Not to be overlooked is the fact that half the presidents over the last 20 years have had medical degrees.

Another noteworthy development has been the establishment of the American Osler Society (AOS) in 1970. Dedicated to sustaining and propagating the intellectual and ethical ideas of Osler, the founding of the AOS was unrelated to any goings on within the AAHM. But while it has provided another public forum for clinician-historians, in so doing, it has probably furthered the growing estrangement of clinicians from the AAHM. Although the AOS has not discouraged the membership of non-M.D.s few have chosen to join. Thus we have the annual spring meetings of both organizations with little crossover in terms of participation although many agree that both groups could profit from a bit of intellectual cross-fertilization. Recently a committee consisting of professional historians and clinicians has been formed and is at work to heal the breach that has developed between the two groups.

Along the way it might be noted that both groups might benefit from a renewed recognition of the importance of linguistic ability in this line of work, especially for those whose efforts are directed to particular segments of medical history. There is a natural tendency to focus on one's own homeland and language and the fading of foreign language skills among English speaking historians and clinicians has probably accented this trend to possible detriment in the quality of the research being reported. Perhaps in recognition of this the English based journal *Medical History* has added "A European Journal for the History of Medicine and Health" to its title as of January 2006 after adding to its editorial board and encouraging colleagues whose first language is not English to contribute.[14]

As such efforts continue it would also be well to remember that it is the quality of the work and not the pedigree of the worker that should be the final arbiter, as the career of Saul Jarcho so abundantly demonstrates.

ACKNOWLEDGMENT: Dr.Thomas G. Benedek kindly made a number of helpful suggestions in reviewing an earlier version of this paper.

REFERENCES

1. Leibowitz JO. *The History of Coronary Heart Disease*. Berkeley & Los Angeles: Univ California Press, 1970.

2. Jarcho S. J.O. Leibowitz. *The History of Coronary Heart Disease* (Review)," *Bull Hist Med* 1972; 46:412-414.

3. Jarcho S. An abbreviated account . *J Pub Health/Bull NY Acad Med* 1988;75(1):89- 97

4. Brush CE, II, Osler at Johns Hopkins, 1899-1905. *The Oslerian* 2004; 5(3):3-5.

5. Bender T, Katz PM, Palmer C and Committee on Graduate Education of the American Historical Association, *The Education of Historians for the Twenty-first Century*. Urbana: Univ of Illinois Press, 2004.

6. DeKruif P. *Microbe Hunters*. New York: Harcourt, Brace & World, 1926.

7. Weisse AB, "Books doctors read. *Hosp Practice* 1993;28(10):68-72, 75-76.

8. Miller G, "The missing seal or highlights of the first half century of the American Association for the History of Medicine. *Bull Hist Med* 1976;50(1):93-121 .

9. ibid p.114

10. Hudson RP. Medical history without medicine. *The Pharos of Alpha Omega Alpha* 2004;67(1):10-11

11. Weisse AB, "Certification/Recertification: self-improvement, self-delusion or self-strangulation. *Persp Med & Biol* 1998;*41:579-590.*

12. Temkin O, *On Second Thought and Other Essays in the History of Medicine and Science*. Baltimore: Johns Hopkins Univ. Press, 2002, p. 11.

13. Burnham JC.A brief history of medical practitioners and professional historians as writers of medical history. *Health and History* 1999;1:250-273.

14. Editorial, *Medical History* 2006;50:1-2.

7

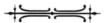

NAMES

I MUST CONFESS TO A lifelong fascination with the matching of names with occupations. Perhaps I first began these associations in medicine when, as a pre-medical student, I worked at some menial position in the posh Harkness Pavilion at New York's Columbia-Presbyterian Medical Center. One day I delivered a package to the office of one, Fordyce B. St. John, M.D., and was "hooked." Perhaps you do not recognize the name of Fordyce B. St. John. Need you? Need anyone? Au contraire. The infant christened Fordyce B. St. John (say it aloud- it is even more impressive when rolled off the tongue like an announced arrival at a royal ball) was predestined for nothing other than the medical profession. And within that profession only the most exclusive type of medical practice. Had an accident of birth placed Fordyce B. St. John three thousand miles eastward it would have been Harley Street in London rather than Fort Washington Avenue in New York that felt his presence.

Forget for the moment the stale my-son-the-doctor jokes and visualize, if you will, the image of his mother presiding over the bassinet of Fordyce B. St. John on an afternoon in the late nineteenth century. Picture her solemnly acknowledging the respects of the supplicants filing by and responding, "Yes. Dr. St. John, I expect, will be prepared to receive you in approximately twenty-two years. Just leave your name at the door."

One might be struck by the fact that so many of the eminent Dock family ultimately became "docs" indeed. You might even smile at the congruence of the father and son osteopathic practice of the Drs. Backrach. But the name Fordyce B. St. John, M.D. allows for no levity. You do not giggle at an apotheosis.

Of course the seeming accident of names and notability is not limited to medicine. It may occur in other professions and probably even surpassed when we come to professional baseball. Recall, for example, that once master of the mound, Rollie Fingers or the murderously competitive Enos Slaughter. Let the old-timers among you reach even further back into the past and come up with the holder of the all-time American League batting record for a single season, .442 in 1901. Who should hold it but the irrepressible Napoleon Lajoie? Finally, who but the moguls of professional baseball could unblinkingly include on one of their rosters a scout going by the name of Clyde Klutz? (Although a more recent pitcher by the name of Putz might be an equally remarkable candidate.)

Such devastating and riotous pairings of people with their profession could be considered a hallmark of our national sport, but my own parochial interests provoked a similar attempt to find them in medicine. The existence of the various medical specialties and the tendency toward group practice provided me with the opportunity to organize some constellations of talent by referring to the Directory of Medical Specialists. I t turns out that in medicine there may be at work some subconscious drive that channels certain physicians into their particular type of practice.

For example, in orthopedic surgery, without any difficulty at all, I was able to "organize" the following group: Drs. Sledge, Harder, Stone, Setter, Rockey, Ribbe, Rust and Hacker. Perhaps slightly more fastidious patients might prefer visiting the offices of Staples, Stover, Stitch, Nettles, Popp, Cram and Flicker. On a more exotic note we have Drs. King, Kang and Kong. But if you broach no sort of nonsense perhaps you would be better off with Drs. Power, House and Sturdy.

The team of Luckey, Sinning and Archdeacon might strike the proper tone for bone-setting if you have a mishap on the ski slope. Perhaps you would be more inclined towards the team of Allgood, Pardon, Comfort and Hope. One pairing that did not have to be made up, incidentally, were two orthopedic surgeons sharing the same address in Merced, California: Drs. Eager and Bever.

Pediatricians likewise seem to cling together by their surnames. One such grouping would include Drs. Wee, Small, Darling, Cuti and Bybee. Imagine one of those typical waiting rooms filled with cheerful paintings of fairy tale characters or Walt Disney cartoon types and then the joy of carting your little tykes into either Dr. Breer, Fox, Stork, Swan, Sparrow or Bearman. More high-minded parents might prefer the offices of Pray, High, Virtue, Elegant, Popish, Upchurch, Rector and Heavenrich. For those parents who are constantly forgetting the names of their pediatrician the office of Drs. Go, Ho, So, Co, Doe, Lo, Mo and No might guarantee the recalling at least the only vowel involved. For the economy-minded we have Drs. Free and Provisor. For those seeking simple or immediate results: Drs. DosRemedios and Miracle.

If your children are easily frightened by men or women in white then take them to the offices of Heaps, Kinder, Bright, Jolly, Hale, Hug, Gay, Sunshine, Merriman and Laughmiller. If, on the other hand, they tend to be intimidated by nothing or no one turn them over to Drs. Kidd, Tamer and Shaver. It that fails you may wish to impress them with the services of the Teutons Kochenderfer, Heffelfinger, Liebschutz, Schimmelpfennig, Etzenhauser and Brunchwyler.

A proctologist once confided to me that deep down, underneath his somewhat offensive exterior lay his basic motivation, the search for the ultimate truth. The rectal surgeons Drs. Furtherer and Ponce de Leon might sympathize with this sort of self image, I imagine. The use of a name that probably produced the most amusement over the years, however, was that of a urologist who advised prospective patients, "If you can't tinkle, call Finkle."

Of all the medical specialties, Obstetrics and Gynecology provides one of the most fruitful (pun intended) for name-gaming. What is more descriptive of what these surgeons do but that proclaimed by Drs. Hacker, Wacker, Packer and Winch? Or Thresher, Messer, Plows and Tinker? Or Reamy, Filler, Calk, Daub and Putterman? Or Bottomy, Bulger, Shearer and Brander?

If the absolute frenzy of activity implied by the above sets your teeth on edge you might at least prefer them to the team of Diddle, Stall, Panic and Groseclose. And you may take comfort that while we do have Drs. Good, Besser and Best among these specialists, we do not have Drs. Bad, Worse and Worst. Ob-Gyn is frequently, after all, a good and bloody business (Drs. Goodspeed, Goodhue, Youngblood, Trueblood and Bloodgood). And it is axiomatic therefore that women should come to look upon their gynecologists only in the most favorable light (see Drs Divine, Loving, Darling and Paalman; also Drs. Warm, Noble, Winner, Polite and Smiley; or for those with more folksy predilections: Drs. Bubala, Gootnick and Gasser). Yet it is difficult to avoid completely the possibilities for conflict (Drs. Fangman, Bitterman, Worsoncraft, Tart, Touchy and Hurt) or, in these times of the shrinking dollar the merest suggestion of avarice (Drs. Much, Price, Fee, Cashman, Talley, Philpott, Roller, Cheatham and Crook).

Anesthesiologists are responsible for administering medication in preparation for surgery or gas mixtures during operations. It seems only fitting therefore to pair Drs. Butman and Backup on the one hand while combining Drs. Given, Mix and Turndorf on the other.

"What," people often ask, "do dermatologists really ever accomplish?"

There would be no room for doubt in the offices of Mopper, Repetto, Slinger and Ditto; nor those of Kinder, Drowns and Dereamer either for that matter. For plastic surgery we offer either Drs. Lucid and Loverme or the confidence inspiring team of Weybright, Weatherly-White and Thoroughgood.

If some neurosurgeon is about to poke around your brain you would perhaps not be too encouraged by the services offered at Mudd, Freshwater and Faeth, and even less assured by the card of Blinderman, Bickers and Trembly. The team of Heifetz and Silvernail, however, has an obvious ring of authority but to go a step further nothing else in medicine approaches baseball in simplicity and totality of expressed expertise as the full names of two others: Doctors Stanley Stellar and Murray Mitts.

- and some favorite titles and authors:
- *Clinical Neurology* by Sir Russell Brain
- *Surgical Diseases of the Chest* by Brian B. Blades, M.D.
- *The Decline of American Gentility* by Stow Persons
- *Manual on Artificial Organs* by Yukihiko Nose
- *Obesity: Causes, Consequences and Treatment* by Louis Lasagna, M.D.

8

DRAWING THE LINE

IMAGINE FOR A MINUTE, if you will, that in 1943 in Auschwitz Josef Mengele had performed the first successful kidney transplantation in humans. This would not be as inconceivable as it may initially appear. In the first decade of the twentieth century the great Franco-American surgeon Alexis Carrel had already devised the proper techniques for the suturing of blood vessels and had even attempted various transplants including that of the kidney in the dog. The main obstacle to transplantation of organs, the rejection of foreign tissues, could easily have been avoided by Mengele who, from his sequestered population of twins could have selected an identical pair for the experiment. At surgery the mechanics of the operation would have been relatively straightforward: remove the two kidneys of the first twin; then remove one kidney from the other and place it in the sibling.

Would such an accomplishment have been hailed as one of the greatest benefits to mankind as it later was in 1990 when Boston surgeon Joseph Murray shared the Nobel Prize in Physiology or Medicine for such a feat performed in 1954? At that time he and his team obtained a normal kidney from one of two brothers, identical twins, and transplanted it into the other who was dying of chronic renal failure. Both young men survived the surgery with the recipient living a relatively normal life for eight years after which the kidney disease recurred in the transplanted organ.

Given the ghoulish nature of Mengele's other experiments upon his hapless victims there would never be any question about denying him this honor for a deed performed under the most criminal of circumstances. This hypothetical black and white case against Mengele is raised only to point out that oftentimes such questions arise in various shades of gray. A number of Hitler's concentration camp doctors, who performed unconscionable medical acts upon Jews and other prisoners, lamely asserted at their trials that these were ethical attempts at serious scientific research for the benefit of mankind. Even when some shred of evidence could be obtained demonstrating a meaningful bit of scientific data, the methods by which they were obtained exempted them from any type of special consideration.

Sadly many Nazi war criminals, including Hitler's doctors, either escaped trial or, after having been convicted and sent to prison, were released early once the initial furor over their misdeeds had subsided and the threat of Soviet imperialism had raised its head. However, given the nature of their crimes and the claims made in their defense, the question arises whether or not any good that may arise from an evil source can ultimately be separated from it.

Consideration of this arose for the author during a review of recent writings about the growth of Yale Medical School as a major academic center in the years following World War I. At that time the school's buildings were literally an assortment of shacks; the hospital was totally outdated; the student enrollment was falling. In 1920 a pathologist from Johns Hopkins, Milton C. Winternitz (1885-1959) was appointed dean, a post he held for the next fifteen years. During this time his efforts to recruit top researchers as faculty, fund the construction of new buildings and generally raise the academic standards of the institution made it, in the judgment of most observers, the outstanding institution it has become.

During this same period fears arose at many American medical schools that a disproportionate number of less desirable students were entering the freshman class, most notably Jews. Quotas began to be established to reverse this trend. When Winternitz's contributions to Yale have been reviewed, oftentimes this aspect of his deanship is either omitted or understated. Admiring apologists for Winternitz have suggested that he was just going along with the trend of the times. Those of us who suffered discrimination during this grim period might take a less charitable view of this admissions officer. Rather than just march in step with this policy, Winternitz led the charge at Yale. The behavior of this Jewish anti-Semite often bordered on the bizarre and at first, he insisted on reviewing all such applicants personally to weed out as many Jews as possible.

In one reported incident a Jewish student with outstanding credentials appeared before him for an interview. The young man's somewhat swarthy appearance prompted the dean to say, "It's bad enough being a Jew, but being a Jew and looking like a nigger is even worse. Go elsewhere!" He did and in later years became a distinguished professor of medicine.

Later on, when the task became too burdensome for Winternitz, he appointed a committee on admissions with strict instructions to accept no more than five Jews and two Italian Catholics. Blacks were completely excluded as were women.

Winternitz lost the deanship not because of his admissions policies but because the faculty rose up against him because of his dictatorial style. He remained at Yale however as a distinguished professor of pathology until 1950. The most ironic aspect of all this is that Winternitz, with his love of learning and intellectual rigor, was, in the final analysis, the quintessential Jew.

In the wake of that horror of horrors, the Holocaust, does the simple limitation on the number of Jews admitted to American medical schools merit such concern? Perhaps when it is recalled that the steps leading to that abomination were incremental. The gas chambers and the ovens did not spring up in a vacuum. First people were deprived of their livelihood; then of their liberty; and finally of their very existence.

The unpredictable and arbitrary ways in which different societies have dealt with judging these acts in the post-war period have been instructive, most strikingly in professions other than medicine.

Following World War II the American poet and fascist sympathizer Ezra Pound was declared a lunatic and placed in an insane asylum. In Norway the 1920 Nobel laureate in literature, Knut Hamsun, welcomed the Nazi takeover of his country and even sent his Nobel Prize to Joseph Goebbels in appreciation. After the war he was fined heavily and shunned until his death in 1952. In 2009, however, the Norwegians celebrated the 150th anniversary of his birth with an emphasis not on the man but the literary accomplishments of his youth which, it must be admitted, were notably free of any Nazi taint.

During the last half-century it seems that in the musical field, especially, reminders of the Nazi era have been dealt with inconsistently. The apolitical Norwegian soprano Kirsten Flagstad had the misfortune to be married to Henry Johansen, an associate of the Nazi puppet Vikun Quisling, who gave his name to the category of traitors and collaborators. Quisling was ultimately executed after being tried for treason. Johanson died while in prison awaiting trial. At the start of the war at her husband's urgent request to return to Europe Flagstad returned to Sweden but refused to sing in any country occupied by the Germans. Following the war, because of her marriage to Johansen , her initial attempts to return to the United States were thwarted and her later engagement at the Metropolitan Opera severely criticized. During this period another soprano, Elisabeth Schwarzkopf, who established herself professionally in Germany during the Nazi period and was a party member, continued to enjoy an uninterrupted international career following the war although boycotted in the United States for several years. Before she died at the age of 90 in 2006 she was made a Dame of the British Empire.

The conductor Wilhelm Furtwängler, who made no secret of his personal distaste for the National Socialists, attempted to help Jewish colleagues escape from their claws. Although he continued to conduct in Berlin during the Nazi period, toward the end of the war he had to flee to Switzerland for his personal safety. He was subjected to severe judgment at a denazification trial after the defeat of Germany and an offer to conduct the Chicago Symphony Orchestra was withdrawn in 1949 after public protest. The treatment of another conductor, the Austrian Herbert von Karajan, was quite different. Karajan had joined the party as early as 1933 and maintained this association throughout the war. Nevertheless, he continued his meteoric rise thereafter serving at the helm of the Berlin Philharmonic for 35 years and gaining recognition as one of the world's outstanding conductors.

Although it was a potent force in German culture before the advent of the Nazis, the music of Richard Wagner became even more so after the seizure of power by Hitler. Nordic mythology as depicted in the Ring cycle seemed to be right in tune with the racial theories of the Nazis and most of the Wagner family became ardent supporters. For music lovers as well as music scholars the less than admirable qualities of the composer have always been acknowledged. Wagner was a notorious scrounger who often rewarded his friends and benefactors by discarding them while, on occasion, stealing the affections of their wives as well. He also made no secret of his anti-Semitism which he advertised in his book, *The Jew in Music,* in which he claimed, Mendelssohn notwithstanding, that Jews were constitutionally incapable of producing great music. Yet the librettos of his operas reveal none of this unless, as some scholars have suggested, you count Klingsor, the evil magician of *Parsifal,* as a Jewish representation. For the most part Wagner's plots are fairy tales with a generous lacing of gobbledygook and dollops of mumbo jumbo and no intelligent person could be expected to take them seriously.

Of course it is the glorious music that redeems Wagner's work from the stories that accompany it and for most of us music lovers it is a compromise we are willing to make. In Israel, however, a non-official ban on the performing of Wagner persists. Inexplicably the music of Carl Orff (1895-1982) continues to be played without protest despite his Nazi associations. After the war Orff falsely claimed to be a member of the anti-Nazi movement in Germany while, in truth, he was a strong supporter of the regime and refused even to try helping an old friend escape execution when he was condemned to death for just such activity.

Where does medicine fit in with all of this? The works produced by the artist—visual, musical or literary—can be described as abstract. There is nothing abstract about a coronary thrombosis, a stroke, a rapidly growing cancer or a human life. Some of us would contend that the calling of medicine is closer to that of the clergy than to those other endeavors; for us the bar must be set higher.

Nothing in the history of anti-Semitism has ever matched the brutality and extent of the Nazi period. But it sprang from a long history of other actions against the Jews, the kind of prejudice that some may be tempted to minimize. Bernhard Schlink, the author of *The Reader,* whose main character is a woman who formerly served as a concentration camp guard, is a non-Jew and a German. He has emphasized that it is important to continue to write about this period to keep alive the memories of the Nazi period. It may be debated as to how much guilt should be shared and by whom but there is no question about bearing the responsibility of remembrance in hopes that such horrors may not recur.

I continue to be haunted by an inscription found on a Parisian monument to the victims of the Holocaust: words to the effect that sometimes we might forgive but we must never forget.

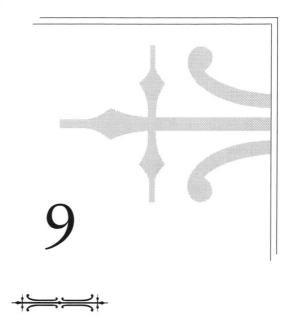

9

THE FIRST HEART OPERATION: THE SURGICAL TREATMENT OF MITRAL STENOSIS

OF ALL THE VARIOUS types of surgery perhaps the one most resisted by the medical establishment in the past was that related to surgery involving the heart. Despite such resistance, by the mid 1940s successful surgical procedures had been introduced to remove diseased pericardium (pericardiectomy) and several procedures performed on the great vessels leading from the heart for the correction or alleviation of such entities as persistent ductus arteriosus, coarctation of the aorta and cyanotic congenital heart disease ("blue babies) (Figure 9.1). Among all these procedures only the repair of traumatic heart lacerations actually involved the heart directly, but this was a desperate act, a life saving spur-of-the-moment effort to rescue patients with otherwise normal hearts from imminent exsanguination.

Rheumatic heart valve disease may occur in some patients following one or more attacks of rheumatic fever. As a result of this damage to the valve, it may not be able to open adequately (stenosis) or it may leak upon attempting to close causing a leaking of blood backward (regurgitation). Any one of the four heart valves may be affected by either of these processes but the most common combination to occur involves stenosis of the mitral valve (MS) causing inadequate emptying of the left atrium into the left ventricle. Pressure in the left atrium builds up proximal to the partially obstructed mitral valve and begins to congest the lungs. It was only the surgical approach to mitral stenosis (MS) that for the first time involved the application of surgical techniques electively to a well-established chronic pre-existing structural abnormality within the heart.

The best documented evidence for serious consideration of surgery for MS

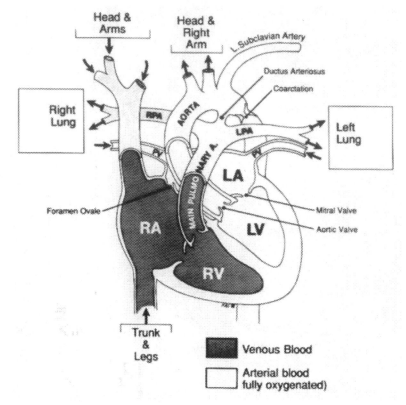

Figure 9.1. – *The heart and major vessels. The human heart is essentially a four-chambered pump. The two chambers on the right, called the right atrium and right ventricle receive dark red (venous) blood from which much of the oxygen has been removed during its course through the body. From the right side of the heart the blood is pumped via the pulmonary artery to the lungs for oxygenation and then via the pulmonary veins it reaches the left side of the heart, the left atrium and ventricle. This bright red blood, now containing its full complement of oxygen is ejected by the left ventricle into the aorta and then, from the vessels arising from it, throughout the body. Valves located strategically within the heart prevent the blood from flowing backwards when the ventricles contract, the tricuspid valve preventing this occurring between the right ventricle and right atrium; the mitral valve performing the same function on the left side of the heart. With each contraction of the ventricles blood passes into a major blood vessel, the pulmonary artery on the right side of the heart and the aorta on the left. As the ventricles relax after each contraction , a set of valves prevent backflow into the right ventricle (the pulmonary valve) and the left ventricle (the aortic valve),*

In the figure a persistently patent ductus arteriosus is shown as well as the location of an abnormal aortic narrowing or coarctation . Abbreviations: RA= right atrium; RV= right ventricle; LA= left atrium; LV= left ventricle; RPA= right pulmonary artery; LPA= left pulmonary artery; PV = pulmonary vein.

appeared as 2 brief letters to the editor of the British journal *The Lancet* around the turn of the century. The first, in 1898, was a communication from D.W. Samways of Cambridge.[1] It concerned "cardiac peristalsis" and dealt mainly with the coordination of atrial and ventricular contractions, emphasizing the importance of the former, especially in mitral valve disease. His concluding sentence: "I anticipate that with the progress of cardiac surgery, some of the severest cases of mitral stenosis will be relieved by slightly notching the mitral orifice and trusting the auricle to continue its defence."

Four years later in 1902 a distinguished physician at St. Bartholomew's Hospital, Sir Lauder Brunton, published a one page article entitled, "Preliminary Note on the Possibility of Treating Mitral Stenosis by Surgical Methods."[2] Obviously distressed by the terminal agonies of his patients with MS, Brunton suggested that they might prefer the option of even a highly risky surgical procedure to continuing on in such a desperate state. Amazingly, within the confines of a single page, Brunton covered essentially all the problems that would later challenge future pioneers in this effort. He, himself, had started animal work and urged others to do the same. He addressed the question of whether to attempt elongation of the mitral opening by cutting medially and then laterally through the pre-existing line of contact between the two valve leaflets, the commissures, or at the middle of the small opening at right angles to the line of closure along the diseased valve cusps (Figure 9.2). He mentioned the possible designs of instruments to carry out the procedure. He offered the options of approaching the valve upward through the left ventricle or downward through a left atrial incision. Perhaps most significant of all, he noted his astonishment at how well the animal hearts he observed managed to keep beating despite all his manipulations.

Judging from the response in *The Lancet* editorial columns that followed, all Brunton ever received for his pains was grief.[3] An unsigned editorial the following week chided him for asking others to perform the research he had started and was obligated to complete. It challenged the ability to perform such a difficult procedure in patients. Even if widening of the valve was achieved, the anonymous author asked, what of "the great tendency" for the edges to re-approximate leaving the situation worse off than before? Similar strictures in the urethra and rectum could be kept open by repeated dilatations but this certainly could not be done for a heart valve.

One letter from a surgeon, Arbuthnot Lane, reported that he had suggested essentially the same approach to a physician, Lauriston Shaw years earlier but the patient had never been referred. A later communication from Shaw placed the episode at least 12 years earlier and defended his decision not to submit the patient to surgery. ("It is possible to do many things that are useless and some things that are harmful.")

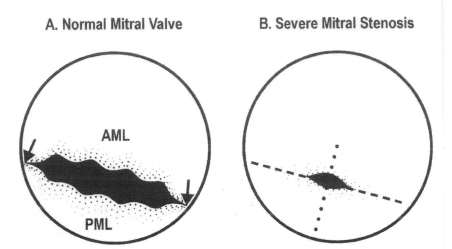

A. Normal Mitral Valve

B. Severe Mitral Stenosis

Figure 9.2. – *Diagrammatic representation of the view looking downward from the left atrial aspect on a normal mitral valve (opening 4-6 cm²) and into the funnel-shaped severely stenotic mitral valve with a typical "fish mouth" opening (1.0 cm² or less). AML= anterior mitral leaflet; PML=posterior mitral leaflet; arrows point to medial and lateral commissures of the valve; dashed lines indicate desired intent of opening obtained by mitral commissurotomy; dotted lines indicate location of "right angle" or transverse cuts across the diseased valve initially attempted in some cases but later discarded.*

This great reluctance to open up the stenotic mitral valve was grounded in the belief that the problem in MS was not valvular obstruction but the failure of the ventricular myocardium to perform normally. This dogma was strongly propounded by none other than the great James Mackenzie (1853-1925) and his successor as the doyen of the British cardiology establishment Sir Thomas Lewis (1881-1945). In the third edition of his text, Mackenzie comments that the size of the narrowed slit in MS found at autopsy did not always correlate with the severity of disease. "Hence, it will be seen that the progress of the disease is largely dependent on the rate of change in the muscle as well as the valve."[4] In the fourth edition he was even more definite on this: "In chronic valvular affections the subjective symptoms of heart failure only arise when exhaustion of the heart muscle sets in."[5] Thomas Lewis in his *Diseases of the Heart* (1937) comments on the surgical failures in MS that had occurred thus far, "... I think they will continue to fail, not only because the interference is too drastic, but because the attempt is based upon what, usually at all events, is an erroneous idea, namely that the valve is the chief source of the trouble."[6]

Both Mackenzie and Lewis may have also focused on the myocardial aspect of rheumatic heart disease as a result of Ludwig Aschoff's discovery in 1904 of the "peculiar nodules" specific to rheumatic carditis and very common in that disease.[7] Arthur Hollman, a student of Lewis and his biographer comments on this at greater length.[8]

Despite the misgivings of the experts there were a number of investigators who, following Brunton's lead, sought to develop a proper animal model for MS, usually the dog, for working out the details of such procedures. None other than Harvey Cushing, the future father of neurosurgery, while still at The Johns Hopkins Hospital worked on this and was succeeded in this effort by B.M. Bernheim and other Americans.[9] While it was relatively easy to create regurgitant lesions with the use of hooks and blades introduced blindly to disrupt the valves under study, the creation of MS eluded them. Even as late as 1929 when John Powers, using electrocautery on the mitral valve with superimposed streptococcal infection, was able to create bulky vegetations that obstructed the valve, the success rate was low and not really a good model for rheumatic MS as found in patients.[10] The end result of such failures was that the animal model for the surgical relief of MS would have to be a human one.

An interesting technical development to these experimental efforts was the development of an instrument by Duff S. Allen and Evarts A. Graham of St. Louis in 1922 that might enable surgeons actually to visualize the valve at surgery before opening it up without having to rely on blind attempts by simply feeling their way.[11] Their cardioscope consisted of a tube like instrument with a small electric bulb at the end through which the operator could observe the structure in contact with it along with a cutting device to open up the valve. Its use with insertions into the left ventricle of dogs was disastrous but the instrument was well tolerated when the left atrium was the portal of entry with several dogs surviving for some time. With the single severely ill patient sent to them for surgery, death occurred intraoperatively even before their cardioscope could be introduced. There were no more referrals.

The first successful surgery for the relief of MS was performed by Elliot C. Cutler at the Peter Bent Brigham Hospital in Boston on May 20, 1923. Cardiologist Samuel A. Levine, who stood by him was co-author on the report that resulted.[12] The patient was a severely symptomatic 12 year-old girl with frequent attacks of hemoptysis. The operation was performed blindly with the approach to the valve through the left ventricle with the cutting instrument, a valvulotome. The patient survived for four and a half years with some evidence of improvement for most of this time. A post-mortem revealed that the surgery had indeed succeeded in partially opening up the diseased mitral valve.

It is important to note the name of the cardiologist on the paper. Without Levine's support and that of the original referring physician the procedure would never have taken place. Another significant inclusion in the introductory part of the paper is mention of the presence of Karl Wenckebach, a world famous Dutch cardiologist from Vienna, as a visitor to the Brigham at the time of surgery. Noted is his "great enthusiasm and approval of the method of attack of the problem that he manifested." This was, after all, at a time when American medicine had not reached its preeminent status and American physicians, especially those aspiring to academic careers, still traveled to Europe for training and guidance. Cutler needed all the medical support he could get. When Levine, who had worked with Mackenzie and Lewis in England during the Great War, had the temerity to send a copy of their paper to Mackenzie his old idol responded, "What a foolish thing you have done. It doesn't matter that the patient lived. You, of all physicians, should know that patients with mitral stenosis are in trouble primarily because of their sick myocardium and not because of the narrowed valve orifice."[13]

Progress in Europe thus far had not been impressive. In 1913 the French surgeon Eugène Doyen described the use of a tenotome (cutting instrument) in a young woman to relieve a muscular obstruction in the right ventricular outflow tract (infundibular pulmonic stenosis) but the patient died postoperatively.[14] In this brief report, however, he also stated he was prepared to tackle mitral stenosis but before he could do this World War I intervened and he was killed in 1916.

In England, despite the predominating animus against mitral surgery Henry Souttar performed the second successful surgery for MS on May 6, 1925, almost 2 years to the day after the Cutler operation.[15] There were some differences in patient selection and technique employed. Souttar's patient, a severely ill 15 year-old girl had a combination of mitral stenosis and regurgitation rather than pure MS. To open the valve Souttar used the left atrial approach rather than that through the left ventricle. This proved to be the favored one as closed heart surgery for MS developed. Finally, although Souttar was prepared to use a cutting instrument to incise the anterior leaflet of the valve, after he palpated the opening with his finger he was able to enlarge the opening digitally with no need for insertion of a blade. During surgery there was a tear in the atrial appendage, a complication which was apparently easily repaired. The whole operation took only an hour and the patient survived for several years, finally succumbing from a cerebral embolis, most likely from a thrombus within the left atrium, common among such patients with advanced disease and atrial fibrillation.

This was the only patient on whom Souttar performed this kind of surgery. When Boston surgeon Dwight Harken 36 years later wrote to him to ask why he had not continued in this effort the 93 year-old Souttar, now Sir Henry Souttar, replied:

"Thank you so much for your very kind letter. I did not repeat the operation because I could not get another case. Although my patient made an uninterrupted recovery the Physicians declared it was all nonsense and in fact that the operation was unjustifiable. In fact it is of no use to be ahead of one's time.

The tear in the appendage had no real bearing on the case but I ought to mention it as it was a detail to avoid. It is wonderful to think of the immense series that you have built up and it is a pleasure to think that my little attempt should have opened the way..."[16]

There was another reported European attempt at MS surgery from Germany in 1926 by Bruno Pribram using the Cutler technique.[17] The patient died on the sixth post-operative day.

Meanwhile, back in Boston Cutler's team continued to operate with, unfortunately, disastrous results. After that initial success all five of the next MS patients operated died between 10 hours and 6 days following the procedure. Surgeons elsewhere had no better luck. In 1929 Cutler and Claude Beck published a sad chronicle of failure as they reviewed the ten operations worldwide thus far that had been performed for this condition.[18] Only their first case and that of Souttar could be counted as successes. Although they encouraged further work on this problem they had to admit that "It may seem ... that further attempts are not justified." It was this latter statement that the medical community took to heart and the field of MS surgery entered a period of the doldrums for the next 2 decades.

After World War II new interest arose in pursuing MS surgery. Over time there had been general improvement in surgical techniques and anesthesia. Blood banking methods had matured and antibiotics had appeared. Wars seem to accelerate change and this was probably an element as well. The introduction of cardiac catheterization provided new hemodynamic data, including pressure gradients across obstructed valves that now could not so easily be ignored. A major stimulus to all this activity was the 1946 publication by Dwight Harken of his experience in removing foreign bodies (mostly shrapnel) from in and around the hearts of servicemen referred to him while he was thoracic surgeon at the 160th General Hospital in England.[19] He had operated on a total of 134 patients without a single fatality. Among these, 56 of the foreign bodies extracted were in or close to the heart and 13 were removed from the heart chambers themselves. Such spectacular results clearly demonstrated the ability of the heart – at least the basically normal one – to tolerate operative manipulation without dire results. (Recall Brunton's comment on this.)

Between 1945 and 1948 four different men in four very different locations renewed the attack on the stenotic mitral valve and they succeeded. These were Dwight E. Harken in Boston; Charles P. Bailey in Philadelphia; Horace G. Smithy in Charleston, South Carolina; and Russell C. Brock in London, England.[20-23]

Following his return from the European theater and flush with his success at the removal of bomb fragments, Harken settled in at Harvard's Peter Bent Brigham Hospital in Boston . He soon resumed the work left undone by Cutler two decades earlier. Despite the loss of the first of his initial two patients undergoing surgery in 1947-48 for relief of MS, Harken persevered and by 1951 could report the results in 86 patients, 71 of whom had undergone simple "finger fracture valvuloplasties" without the use of any cutting instrument. About one in four did not survive but this was a great improvement over the outcome in a control group of 19 patients with a similar severity of MS who had refused the operation. Among these 17 were dead one year after the time of referral.[24]

Charles Bailey had the most difficult time of all of these pioneers in promoting the operation ("mitral commissurotomy") to which he had devoted much of his professional life. His travails resulted as much from his highly competitive and prickly personality as from the obstacles he found confronting him. Fortunately, a written transcription of his experiences and beliefs exists to give insight into the motivation of Bailey and others like him.[25] Born in Neptune, New Jersey, at the age of 12 Bailey witnessed his father's death from MS at the age of 42. From this experience grew his determination to find a cure. After graduating from Hahnemann Medical College and completing an internship he spent five years in private practice in Lakewood, New Jersey, before taking additional training in thoracic surgery and returning to Hahnemann in the department of surgery. His first two MS patients, operated on at Hahnemann in 1945 and 1946, both died. In 1948 he attempted a third operation at Memorial Hospital in Wilmington, Delaware. This too failed due to post-operative complications. At Hahnemann the professor of cardiology had called Bailey in to inform him that, as a physician, it was his Hippocratic duty to do no harm when he could not do good. He added that it was his Christian duty to keep Bailey from doing any more of these procedures. Characteristically Bailey replied that he was a victim of "the jury being out before the court had been called into session." He affirmed his belief in this type of surgery when medical treatment for MS was practically worthless. He proclaimed that "... it was *my* Christian duty to continue with this effort and make it successful; and that I was prepared to spend the rest of my life in that effort."

He was soon denied surgical privileges in three of the five hospitals in Philadelphia where he had been on staff and realized that any further failures would completely end any further efforts on his part. With this thought in mind, he scheduled one mitral surgery in the morning at the Philadelphia General Hospital and another for the afternoon at Episcopal Hospital. If the first failed in the morning he would have one more chance in the afternoon before all his privileges had been cut off. Then, at the ripe old age of 38, Bailey contracted measles, necessitating a month's delay in his plans. When the day of judgment finally arrived, the first patient, an elderly man with far advanced MS and many other medical problems, did not survive surgery. However, the second patient at Episcopal Hospital, a woman who was a much better risk, improved significantly. Transverse cutting of the valve was discarded as too likely to result in significant mitral regurgitation post-operatively. The transatrial approach was less provocative of ventricular arrhythmias; perhaps more importantly with the blind procedure required, the transatrial approach made it relatively easy for the surgeon's finger to find the valve opening through the frequently funnel shaped diseased mitral valve. Much less certain was positioning of a cutting or dilating instrument passed upward from the left ventricular apex. Bailey's operative technique, "mitral commissurotomy," which became the standard, involved opening up the stenotic valve along the line of the pre-existing commissures by the surgeon's finger with or without the assistance of a cutting instrument attached to the exploring finger of the surgeon. Years later, when asked about his persistence in the face of the initial failures, Bailey replied:

"Obviously, I felt there were irrelevant reasons for the loss of the first four patients and the principle was entirely sound and could be developed but needed further effort…. Finally, however, you have to face 'the moment of truth' and the poignancy is so great that I can't really express it. You know that almost all the world is against it; you know that you have a great personal stake and might even lose your medical license, or at least your hospital privileges, if you persist. In fact the thought crosses your mind that maybe you really *are* crazy. And yet you feel that it has to be done and it must be right."

Brock at Guy's Hospital in London was gaining increased stature as a skilled heart surgeon as a result of his achievement in relieving pulmonic stenosis associated with Tetralogy of Fallot for the first time with a report of success in three patients.[26] His report of success in six of eight patients with MS brought to surgery added additional luster to his reputation and to the acceptance of this kind of surgery for patients with rheumatic heart disease. The technique used initially was similar to that of Bailey. Later on Brock used a dilating instrument introduced through the left ventricle, guided into place by his finger inserted through the left atrium. This resulted in more complete opening of the stenotic valve.

In terms of "poignancy" the story of the youngest of the group, Horace Smithy stands out most prominently. Working at the Medical College of

South Carolina in Charleston, Smithy, using either the Cutler ventricular approach or the transatrial access to the valve performed eight operations for MS in 1948. Six of these patients survived, a result that encouraged Bailey, when learning of them, to persist in his own efforts. Initially Smithy, as well as Harken, used an instrument to punch a hole in the diseased valve and extract a piece of tissue ("partial valvectomy") partially relieving the MS without causing significant mitral regurgitation. Later they both abandoned this for the "mitral commissurotomy" technique of Bailey.

When Bailey and Smithy first met in person at the conclusion of a surgical meeting, Smithy asked Bailey to listen to his chest. Smithy had severe aortic stenosis, probably on a congenital basis and his outlook was not good. He asked Bailey if he had ever operated on this other valve lesion and he had not, nor had anyone else. (This was before the era of open-heart surgery where any valve could be approached under direct vision.) When Bailey deferred from attempting this, Smithy approached Alfred Blalock of Johns Hopkins who had devised the "blue baby operation" with Helen Taussig. Blalock and Smithy attempted a closed-heart repair in one patient with aortic stenosis who died on the operating table. Blalock could not be persuaded to attempt any more such procedures and Smithy was doomed. He died in 1948, the same year of his achievements in MS at the age of 34.

Remarkably the first successes of 3 of these 4 surgeons, working independently, occurred within a six month period. Smithy's first survivor was operated on Jan. 18,1948; Bailey's on June 10; and Harken's on June 16. Brock's first success came 3 months later on the 16th of September in the same year. Thanks to the combined results of this surgical quadrumvirate the operation for MS was established and would prolong thousands upon thousands of lives in the years to come.

Following the breakthrough with surgery for MS Harken, Brock and Bailey continued to make important contributions to the field of cardiovascular surgery. However, while the first two remained firmly ensconced in their home institutions for the duration of their careers, Bailey, unpredictable as ever, set off in other directions. Alarmed by the rise in medical litigation, he gave up his surgical practice in order to obtain a law degree from Fordham University in 1973. He then joined a firm specializing in physicians' problems. In 1986 he founded a non-profit insurance firm before dying at the age of 82 in 1993 from, of all things, heart valve disease (aortic stenosis).

Closed mitral commissurotomy, important as it was, represented only a first step in the surgical treatment of valve disease and was not applicable to many of those suffering from various other types of valve disease. There were some patients whose primary mitral problem was mitral regurgitation rather than stenosis; some patients had valves that were so heavily calcified that they could not be opened by "finger fracture" with or without cutting instruments; some patients who underwent too vigorous a commissurotomy wound up with severe mitral regurgitation, equally threatening to their welfare. Finally, there were patients with other valve involvement, notably aortic, which required an open-heart approach for correction. After cardiopulmonary by-pass became available in the mid-fifties such problems could now be effectively addressed. Many valves that could not be restored to normal or near normal function by surgical manipulation after open heart exposure could be replaced with the introduction of mechanical prostheses such as the Starr-Edwards ball-cage valve.[27] Bio-prostheses using pig valves or pericardium would become another option.

The invention of the cardiac defibrillator and pacemakers further enhanced the ability of surgeons to work safely on the heart. And advances in catheter and balloon technology have enabled a different approach to opening up stenotic valves as long as they remain pliable. The technique introduced by Kanji Inoue in 1984 involves passing a balloon-tipped catheter from a femoral vein up into the right atrium and across the atrial septum with advancement through the narrowed mitral valve at which point the balloon is inflated to open it up.[28] Results comparable to closed and open mitral commissurotomy have been achieved by this innovative relatively non-invasive technique.[29]

However, the most effective advance in the control of rheumatic heart disease has not been surgical at all. It was found that the valvular disease resulting in some patients suffering attacks of rheumatic fever was the result of an auto-immune reaction in response to an upper respiratory infection with a certain type of streptococcus. With the introduction of long term prophylaxis with sulfa drugs and later penicillin in patients following an attack of rheumatic fever there has been a major decrease in rheumatic fever and rheumatic heart disease among modern industrialized nations. In underdeveloped countries where antiobiotics are rarely readily attainable and heart-lung machines often non-existent, MS remains a common problem. In such places the closed mitral commissurotomy remains an important surgical technique.[30-31] Early fears that the surgically separated diseased valve edges would quickly re-adhere post-operatively have not been realized. Following an adequate procedure a large majority of these MS patients undergoing closed commissurotomy will go for ten years or more before re-operation may be required.[32]

One wonders what Brunton would have made of all this if he were still alive. During his lifetime he received honors and recognition for making one of the most important contributions to the medical treatment of heart disease with the introduction of nitrates (amyl nitrite) for *angina pectoris*. He might have smiled to see that the modest proposal he made in 1902, for which he had received so much disapprobation, had resulted in his earning major credit for one of the greatest surgical advances as well.

REFERENCES:

1. Samways DW. Cardiac peristalsis: Its nature and effects. *The Lancet* 1898;1:927.

2. Brunton L. Preliminary note on the possibility of treating mitral stenosis by surgical methods. *The Lancet* 1902;1:352.

3. Shumacker HB, Jr. *The Evolution of Cardiac Surgery.* Bloomington:Indiana University Press, 1992:33.

4. Mackenzie J. *Diseases of the Heart. Third Edition.* London:Oxford University Press, 1914:333.

5. Mackenzie J. *Diseases of the Heart. Fourth Edition.* London:Oxford University Press, 1925:362.

6. Lewis T. *Diseases of the Heart.* London:MacMillan, 1937:148.

7. Aschoff L. Concerning the question of myocarditis *in* Willius FA, Keys TE. *Classics of Cardiology Vol. 2* Malabar:Krieger, 1983:733-739 (English translation from the original German).

8. Holman A. *Sir Thomas Lewis. Pioneer Cardiologist and Clinical Scientist.* London:Springer, 1997:172-174.

9. Cushing H, Branch JRB. Experimental and clinical notes on chronic valvular lesions in the dog and their possible relation to future surgery of the cardiac valves. *J Med Res* 1908;17:471-486; Bernheim BM. Experimental surgery of the mitral valve. *Johns Hopkins Hosp Bull* 1909;20:107-110; Cutler EC, Levine SA, Beck CC. The surgical treatment of mitral stenosis. Experimental and clinical studies. *Arch Surg* 1924;9:689-821.

10. Powers JH. The experimental production of mitral stenosis. *Arch Surg* 1929;18:1945-1959.

11. Allen DS, Graham EA. Intracardiac surgery – A new method. *JAMA* 1922;79:1028-1030.

12. Cutler EC, Levine SA. Cardiotomy and valvotomy for mitral stenosis. Experimental observations and clinical notes concerning an operated case with recovery. *Bost Med Surg J* 1923;188:1023-1027.

13. Shumacker, *Cardiac Surgery*:39.

14. Doyen E. Chirurgie des malformations congenitales ou acquises du Coeur. *Presse Méd* 1913;21:860.

15. Souttar HS. The surgical treatment of mitral stenosis. *Brit Med J* 1925;2:603-606.

16. A photograph of the entire letter appears in Harkin DE, Curtis LE. Heart Surgery – legend and a long look. *Am J Cardiol* 1967;19:398.

17. Pribram BO. Die Operative Behandling der Mitralstenose. *Arch Clin Chur* 1926;142:458-465.

18. Cutler EC, Beck CS. The present status of the surgical procedures in chronic valvular disease of the heart. *Arch Surg* 1929;18:402-416.

19. Harken DE. Foreign bodies in and in relation to the thoracic blood vessels and heart. *Surg Gynec & Obst* 1946;83:117-125.

20. Harken DE, Ellis LB, Ware PF, Norman LR. The surgical treatment of mitral stenosis. 1. Valvuloplasty. *N Engl J Med* 1948;239:801-809.

21. Bailey CP. The surgical treatment of mitral stenosis (mitral commissurotomy). *Dis Chest* 1949;15:377-397.

22. Smithy HG, Boone JA, Stallworth JM. Surgical treatment of constrictive valvular disease of the heart. *Surg Gynec Obst* 1950;90:175-192.

23. Baker C, Brock RC, Campbell M. Valvotomy for mitral stenosis: report of six successful cases. *Brit Med J* 1950;1:1283-1293.

24. Harken DE, Dexter L, Ellis LB, Farrand RE, Dickenson JF. The surgery of mitral stenosis III. Finger fracture valvuloplasty. *Annals Surg* 1951;134:722-742.

25. Weisse AB. *Conversations in Medicine. The Story of Twentieth-Century American Medicine in the Words of Those Who Created It.* New York:New York University Press, 1984:133-156.

26. Brock RC. Pulmonary valvotomy for the relief of congenital pulmonary stenosis. *Brit Med J* 1948;1:1121-1126.

27. Starr A, Edwards ML. Mitral replacement. Clinical experience with a ball-valve prosthesis. *Annals Surg* 1962;154:726-740.

28. Inoue K, Owaki T, Nakamura T, Mamoto N. Clinical application of transvenous mitral commissurotomy by a new balloon catheter. *J Thor Cardiovasc Surg* 1984;87:394-402.

29. Ben Farhat M, Mokdad A, Betbout F, Gamra H, Jarrar M, Tiss M, Hammami S, Thalbi R, Addad F. Percutaneous balloon versus surgical closed and open mitral commissurotomy. Seven year follow up results of randomized trial. *Circulation* 1998;97:245-250.

30. John S, Bashi VV, Jairaz PS, Muralidharan S. Ravikumar E, Rajarajaswari S, Sukumar IP, Sundar Rao PSS. Closed mitral valvotomy: early results and long term follow-up of 3724 patients. *Circulation* 1983;68: 891-896.

31. Eren E, Samilgil A. Özler A, Ulufer T, Tulpar S. Closed mitral commissurotomy in Istanbul, Turkey. Results in 4403 cases. *Tex Heart Inst J* 1986;13:143-146.

32. Hickey MSJ, Blackstone EH, Kirklin JW, Dean LS. Outcome probabilities and life history after surgical mitral commissurotomy: Implications for balloon commissurotomy. *J Am Coll Cardiol* 1991;17:29-42.

10

ABSOLUTELY THE LAST WORD ON PHYSICAL DIAGNOSIS. NOT!

It is GENERALLY AGREED that the ability to perform a skilled physical examination has become a lost art in modern medicine. The last few generations of newly minted medical graduates have failed to develop the skills that were once considered part and parcel of a competent practitioner. This trend is universally deplored but nothing or no one seems capable of reversing it. Indeed, some of the leaders of medicine in this supertechnical age are beginning to look upon this as a natural development and turning to technological solutions for these human failings.

In no field has this been so apparent as in cardiovascular medicine, a specialty that a half century ago attracted this writer expressly because of the assumed ability of a well-trained cardiologist to arrive at a correct diagnosis in a patient simply by taking a good medical history and performing a thorough physical examination. An electrocardiogram was granted as the only supplement to these other diagnostic modalities. The models of such acquired skill were people like W. Proctor Harvey, Samuel A. Levine and Aubrey Leatham. Their papers and monographs were required reading.[1,2] However, all qualified cardiologists and even seasoned physicians of any stripe, were expected to have superior abilities along these lines and transmit such knowledge to students and residents in training. However, recent studies evaluating these skills among students, house staff and even faculty have shown a 20 to 80 percent error rate in recognizing actual or simulated findings. [3-7]

It seems that our recent medical graduates are more at ease in discussing the splitting of a strand of DNA than that of the second heart sound, the key

95

to differentiating many innocent murmurs from such serious conditions as atrial septal defect, aortic stenosis, pulmonic stenosis, pulmonary hypertension and left bundle-branch block. Innocent or "functional" murmurs are so common among normal children, anemic patients and pregnant women, among others, that they cry out for such differentiation at the bedside or the office. However it seems that such patients too often are sent off for chest films and echocardiograms to compensate for the physician's inadequacy.

In the face of such diagnostic shortfalls some of those responsible for the training of physicians have simply given up and taken the view that the lesser of two evils, depending on machines for diagnosis, is better than having no diagnosis at all. The downside of this, however, is considerable. Although hand-held echocardiograph machines are now available the cost is not negligible. Consider equipping each American graduating class, approaching 20,000 each year now, plus practicing physicians with these devices. Then there is the question of competency among non-cardiologists, trained in this discipline, in interpreting the findings. Regional wall motion abnormalities, the hallmark of coronary heart disease, one of our major health problems, are one of the most difficult of findings to interpret accurately. Small vegetations located on the valves in infective endocarditis may be missed by one not expert in the technique. Missing such findings may work to the harm of the patient by giving a false sense of security to the non-expert examiner just as misinterpretation of normal variants as abnormalities may lead both him and the patient astray.

There is also a cost of unnecessary anxiety to a patient and his family. Besides the not inconsiderable cost of such procedures are the days of doubt wondering whether or not some serious heart disease is present. Of equal importance is the effect of using machinery in further separating doctor and patient in this age of rampant technology. Whatever the medical value of the encounter between any healer and his subject has been, the possible beneficial effect of the contact in itself is not negligible. Although earlier monarchs often used the "royal touch" for scrofula it might be wondered how many of their subjects with what we would now call "psychosomatic ailments" might have benefited from that laying on of hands. The simple performance of the physical examination can constitute a strong tie binding together doctor and patient in our increasingly impersonal medical world.

With the left middle finger pressed against the chest and the other fingers elevated so as not, by contact, to dampen any reflected sound sensations, the left hand adapts a configuration much like that of the classical ballerina's extended hand. In preparation to strike its opposite, the right hand adopts a similar appearance as the middle finger "plexor" repeatedly descends briskly by graceful flicks at the wrist. The exercise becomes almost terpsichorean in character.

With the physician exhibiting intense concentration as he follows this with auscultation over the chest the whole proceeding can be appreciated on a more primitive level. The doctor's percussion represents his tapping on the thoracic "door" to the patient's inner being and with auscultation, his head bent close over the stethoscope, he listens for a reply. The great cardiologist Paul Dudley White used this aspect of the physical examination to great psychological advantage at times when confronted with a severely agitated patient. He might mutter as an encouragement, "The first sound seems just fine." The anxious subject might think to himself, "Well, the first sound is good; perhaps the others are as well."

By gently palpating the abdomen with obvious concern for the patient's sense of well-being the physician can further strengthen that important bond: "Does it hurt here? How about here? Tell me if this bothers you." All this in a tone of concern and sympathy.

The performance of a skilled physical examination involves not merely esthetics and psychology. When evaluated objectively – which is not done too often – it can hold up quite well to critical scrutiny. Splitting of the second heart sound (the audible separation of aortic and pulmonic valve closure) is not a rare, esoteric finding; it can be detected in almost 80 percent of all normal individuals from six to 74 years of age.[8] Enlargement of the left ventricle determined by percussion and palpation correlates well with computed tomography.[9] Although not as reliable as CT scanning, physical examination to detect pleural effusions is comparable to conventional chest radiography.[10] The third heart sound, occurring with filling of the ventricle, detected by experienced physicians matches up well with that recorded by phonocardiography.[11] Even a century and half after Laennec ways have been found to improve upon percussion and auscultation.[12]

Sadly those most capable of passing on these skills to physicians in training have more or less disappeared either as the result of death or retirement. The remaining few, at least in the experience of this writer, who offer such services are politely rebuffed. It is like allowing the few remaining Stradivari and Guarneri remaining to lay about abandoned in some obscure closet, lost to the ears of the world.

The current vogue of using troponins and other biological markers for the diagnosis of congestive heart failure is bewildering to any seasoned physician worth his salt (if you will pardon that word in this context). Although this may be difficult in a patient with long standing lung disease and superimposed cardiac decompensation, in the majority of patients the diagnosis can be made with the exchange of a few words followed by an examination of the neck veins, chest, abdomen and lower extremities.

This all does not mean that emerging clinicians may be forever denied the rewards of such skills. Physical diagnosis is largely self taught. Through constant application and correlation with other objective data any physician can become competent if he or she so wishes or is compelled to do so.

About fifteen years ago at the main general hospital in Nairobi the chief of medicine received a group of American physicians on tour. An ethnic Indian, she was nonetheless a loyal Kenyan who, upon finishing her medical training probably in the United Kingdom, returned home to serve her country. Back in Africa, she found that her hospital could not afford the luxury of routine chest x-rays for use in the diagnosis of chest diseases despite their frequency in that part of the world. As she conducted us through wards filled with sufferers from pulmonary tuberculosis and other chest diseases, she related how she had come to rely on physical diagnosis for her assessment of patients; how she had become quite proficient in this; and how only rarely and in very complicated cases did she feel the need for radiological confirmation.

Such commitment recalls another vignette involving Dr. White. He was listening intently to the chest of a patient referred to him with a heart murmur. The medical resident prematurely inquired, "Dr.White, do you hear the murmur?" White responded tersely, "I am not yet finished with the first heart sound." It is this systematic, intense and unhurried kind of analysis that can reap great diagnostic gains for all who wish to become masters of the art.

And it is the art of medicine that creates bonds, this time not between patient and doctor but between teacher and student. When I was still making ward rounds I always relished being presented with a patient with aortic regurgitation. With a captive audience of students and house staff in tow it was always great fun to indulge in the colorful history of this disease. While pointing out the characteristic murmur of aortic regurgitation I was also sure to include highlighting its other dramatic physical signs: the collapsing water hammer or Corrigan pulse; Quincke's pulse (arterial pulsations visible in the finger nail beds); DeMusset's sign (bobbing of the head after the French literary figure who had the disease); and the diastolic whoosh elicited in addition to the systolic one as the pressure of the stethoscope was adjusted over the femoral artery (Duroziez's sign).

It was not all cardiology in this respect. About once every two or three months we would approach the bedside of a patient who seemed obviously hypothyroid and this had been completely missed by the house staff. Nothing gave one greater joy than to grab a reflex hammer from some unsuspecting tyro and demonstrate the characteristic slow return of the brachial and Achilles reflexes in the myxedematous patient. "Better get some thyroid tests on this patient," I would advise – and often enough I would be right.

REFERENCES

1. Levine SA, Harvey WP. *Clinical Auscultation of the Heart.* Philadelphia: W.B. Saunders, 1949.

2. Leatham A. *Auscultation of the Heart and Phonocardiography.* London: Churchill, 1970.

3. St. Clair EW, Oddone EZ, Waugh RA, et al. Assessing housestaff diagnostic skills using a cardiology patient simulator. *Ann Int Med* 1992;117:751-56.

4. Mangione S, Neiman LZ. Cardiac auscultatory skills of internal medicine and family practice trainees. A comparison of diagnostic proficiency. *J Am Med Assoc* 1997;278:717-22.

5. Roldan CA, Shively BK, Crawford HH. Value of the cardiovascular physical examination for detecting valvular heart disease in asymptomatic subjects. *Am J Cardiol* 1996;77:327-31.

6. March SK, Bedynek JL, Chizner MA. Teaching cardiac auscultation effectiveness of a patient-centered teaching conference on improving cardiac auscultatory skills. *Mayo Clin Proc* 2005;80:1443-48.

7. Vukanovic-Criley JM, Criley S, Warde CM et al. Competency in cardiac examination skills in medical students, trainees, physicians and faculty. *Arch Int Med* 2006;166:610-16.

8. Weisse AB, Schwartz ML, Heinz BS et al. Intensity of the normal second heart sound components in their traditional auscultatory areas. *Am J Med* 1967;43:171-77.

9. Heckerling PS, Wiener SL, Wolfkiel CJ et al. Accuracy and reproducibility of precordial percussion and palpation for detecting increased left ventricular end-diastolic volume and mass. *J Am Med Assoc* 1993;270:1943-48.

10. Diaz-Guzman E, Budev MM. Accuracy of the physical examination in evaluating pleural effusion. *Clev Clinic J Med* 2008;75:297-303.

11. Marcus G, Vessey J, Jordan MV et al. Relationship between accurate auscultation of a clinically useful third heart sound and level of experience. *Arch Int Med* 2006;166:617-22.

12. Guarino JR. Auscultatory percussion, a new aid in the examination of the chest. *J Kansas Med Soc* 1974;193-94.

11

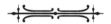

NOBLE, NOT NOBEL: HOW NOT TO WIN THE MOST PRESTIGIOUS PRIZE IN MEDICINE

On A Fateful Day in April 1888 the inventor of dynamite, Alfred Nobel, could peruse one French newspaper and be confronted with his own obituary. What had happened was that the newspaper had mistaken Alfred's death for that of his older brother, Ludwig. What was particularly disturbing about the obituary was that it characterized Alfred as "a merchant of death" who had made his fortune by discovering "new ways to mutilate and kill." This was not the first time that such canards had been leveled at him but, as noted by his biographers, it was a major stimulus among many others leading to the famous will of 1895 establishing the Nobel Prizes.[1]

Who was the real Alfred Nobel? Perhaps a look back on his personal history may provide important clues to answering this question. Much of it involves how he and his brothers were brought into the family business, mainly munitions, by their enterprising but often unsuccessful father, Immanuel.

From the time of his youth Alfred's health was delicate. He suffered rheumatologic symptoms for which, from the age of 20, he was repeatedly sent to spas for rest and recuperation. He was shy and melancholic. He wrote poetry and admired those more proficient in it than himself. His respect for two Norwegian poets, it is believed, prompted his placing the Peace Prize in the hands of Norwegians rather than the Swedes. Largely self-taught, he became a cultured individual fluent in five languages. However his remarks about himself were self-deprecating. In later life he referred to himself as "worm eaten" and "…a misanthrope, but exceedingly benevolent;" "cranky, but a super idealist." He was unlucky in love and connubial bliss eluded him. He died childless. All this is not what one would ordinarily consider typical in a successful industrial titan.

Besides becoming a formidable business man he was a brilliant researcher, and in 1890, five years before his death, he had already been in touch with physiologists from the Karolinska Institute, planning for a research laboratory in Paris. In 1894 he made grants to Ivan Pavlov and another Russian for their research.

What did his will provide for? Among the five prizes awarded, the Peace Prize represented a direct response to the war mongering charges leveled against him. There was then a literary prize and three prizes in science. A prize in economics was added in 1968. Of the three scientific awards it is the prize in medicine that has attracted the most public attention – not because medical discoveries are intrinsically of greater value than those in chemistry or physics but because such achievements are perceived by the medical community and the lay public as well as having a more immediate and comprehensible impact upon our well being. Therefore it is to the Prize in Physiology or Medicine that this paper is directed.

Controversy has come part and parcel with the awards right from the beginning. The controversies have basically involved two questions: 1) Why have certain important medical discoveries been ignored? 2) In the cases of certain discoveries that have been honored why have certain individuals associated with them been excluded? Determining the answers to these questions has not been easy for historians and others. This is in large part due to the history and policies of the Nobel Foundation which, either by default or by design, has obfuscated many of its decisions.

This is not to deny that the Foundation has made some efforts at explaining its operations. In 1951 a book was published describing the events leading up to the will as well as its conditions.[2] For each of the prizes there is also a narrative provided to describe the past 50 years of events written by a Nobel insider, in the case of the medical prize Gören Liljestrand. Second and third editions appeared in 1962 and 1972 with the Liljestrand account revised by Carl Gustaf Bernhard.[3] These accounts provide a few tantalizing nuggets of information about certain disputed choices but they are few and far between. Upon request the Foundation will supply scholars with a copy of the statutes governing its operation.[4] Around 1999 the Foundation began keeping its records in English as well as Swedish for easier access, although this is not to be applied retroactively over the previous century of awards.[5]

On the other hand, certain policies enacted only emphasize the aura of mystery that surrounds the deliberations of the Nobel committees. When a new Swedish law was developed in the 1970s requiring the Karolinska

Institute, among other state organizations, to reveal all such information to the public, a new organization, the Nobel Assembly, was formed in 1977 which would be free of such a requirement.[6] However the greatest obstacle to any inquiry into their operations is the informational blackout on the past 50 years of awards. While it is understandable why the Foundation would wish to shield itself from protest or controversy in this way it makes any research into half the history of the prizes well nigh impossible. For the years prior to 1951 the names of nominees, the basis for nominations and the identity of the nominating individual are available on the internet site. Also available on request by credited researchers are the committee reports commenting on these nominations. However, for both successful and unsuccessful nominations no written records have been kept of all the discussions pertinent to the selection or rejection of each discovery or those who may or may not have been credited with contributing to it. Why was one discovery chosen over another?

Why was this individual included in the prize and not another? The answers to such questions can only remain a matter of conjecture in the absence of written documentation.

In order to gain insight into the basis of such decisions it was decided to approach the problem in two ways: subjecting the wording of the will to careful scrutiny to determine to the best of our ability the intent of the author; and providing some examples of the types of discoveries that have been rejected as well as the characteristics of those individuals, often outstanding in their fields, who were excluded from sharing the prize with others. To assist in this assessment, biographies of Nobel and a number of works devoted to the history of the Nobel Prize were consulted.[7]

The Will and the Way

The will was written without the aid of lawyers whom Nobel distrusted. He left the carrying out of its provisions to two executors. One of these was a young engineer, Rognar Sohlman, his personal assistant during the last three years of his life and later a biographer. The will was short and to the point. Nonetheless, certain provisions (highlighted below) have required specific interpretations, some of which have led to controversy. After a few small bequests the pertinent part of the will reads as follows:

> The whole of my remaining realizable estate shall be dealt with in the following way: the capital, invested in safe securities by my executors, shall constitute a fund, the interest on which shall be annually distributed in the form of prizes to **those who, in the preceding year, have conferred**

106 | *Allen B. Weisse, M.D.*

the greatest benefit to mankind. The said interest shall be divided into five equal parts, which shall be apportioned as follows: one part to the person who shall have made the most important discovery or **invention** within the field of physics; one part to the person who shall have made the most important chemical discovery or improvement; **one part to the person who shall have made the most important discovery within the domain of physiology or medicine;** one part to the person who shall have produced in the field of literature the most outstanding work in an ideal direction; and one part to the person who shall have done the most or best work for fraternity between nations, for the abolition or reduction of standing armies and for the holding and promotion of peace congresses. The prize for physics and chemistry shall be awarded by the Swedish Academy of Sciences; that for physiological or medical works by the Caroline Institute in Stockholm; that for literature by the Academy in Stockholm and for champions of peace by a committee of five persons to be elected by the Norwegian Storting. It is my express wish that in awarding the prizes **no consideration whatever shall be given to the nationality of the candidates,** but that the most worthy shall receive the prize, whether he be a Scandinavian or not.

Referring to the will one might ask about the specification of "physiology **or** medicine." The account by Göran Liljestrand sheds considerable light on this.[8] In 1890 a member of the Karolinska Institute by the name of von Hofson had a brief conversation with Alfred Nobel while visiting Paris, a favorite residence of the peripatetic industrialist. Dr. von Hofson wrote about this meeting to a colleague at the Karolinska, a physiologist by the name of J.E. Johannson. He wrote with enthusiasm about Nobel's interest: "On this occasion we discussed some physiological and biological ideas which appealed strongly to his inventive and inquiring mind. In that connection he expressed his sincere wish to become acquainted with some young, well-trained Swedish physiologist with whom he could work, or rather, who might be able to carry out some of the many original and ingenious ideas on the subject of physiology that were germinating in his highly inventive brain." This resulted that same year in Johannson's visit to Nobel in Paris, where he remained for five months during which time Nobel made plans for setting up a medical institute for such research in the French capitol. After all, Nobel was an experimentalist himself. He was no doubt aware of prominent research institutes in Europe such as those in Paris, Breslau, Berlin and Leipzig.

In 1894 shortly before his death Nobel contributed funds to laboratories headed by I.P. Pavlov (later Nobel laureate in 1904) and another Russian scientist.

Thus, to the modern mind, the somewhat odd appearance of "physiology" in association with "medicine" in designating the prize becomes clear in this context. What one might also assume is that by identifying two sides of this coin as he did, Nobel was separating out the laboratory work that might result in a great discovery from the clinical gains at the bedside that might also represent "the greatest benefit to mankind." In practice, however, especially in recent years, it has been the accomplishments of laboratory medicine rather than those in the clinics or beyond that have received the most recognition in Stockholm.

Specifying "the preceding year" most likely reflected Nobel's desire to stimulate and support new research coming from relative newcomers to the field of physiological or medical research. By focusing the award with its considerable financial component on the young, Nobel clearly intended that lack of funds not preclude further achievements by such junior scientists in the future. Although this may have been a major consideration at the time the awards were instituted, today, with the much greater access of investigators to government and foundation support, this is a much less urgent concern. Additionally it soon became apparent that it might take more than a year for a major discovery to be recognized. The interpretation of "preceding year" soon came to include *recognition* of a discovery within the preceding year with many of the awards given for important insights and discoveries made decades or more before. Along the lines of favoring future productivity among the young and active, however, the Nobel Foundation in Article 4 of its statutes prohibits awarding the prizes posthumously.

With this as a background, one can sift through whatever evidence is available from existing publications, available Nobel Foundation documents, the investigations of others seeking explanations about the workings of the Foundation, and one's own knowledge base about the history of medicine to offer a number of possible explanations as to why certain discoveries have been ignored and why many worthy medical scientists never seemed worthy enough in Stockholm.

HOW NOT TO WIN

Correct or relate to a previous error in the awarding of the prize

The selection committees of the Nobel Foundation have rarely made major blunders in their choice of prize winners. One involved the award in 1927 to Julius Wagner-Jauregg for the fever treatment of neurosyphilis by the introduction of malarial parasites into the blood streams of patients. In 1949 the award went to Antonio Egas Moniz for lobotomy in the treatment of mental disease, another striking example of such misjudgments. However neither had such a wide-reaching effect on the subsequent conduct of the committees as their misguided award in 1926 to Johannes Fibiger for the "discovery of *Spiroptera carcinoma*."

Fibiger, a highly respected Danish pathologist, reported that in rats gastric cancer could be caused by a type of worm that had invaded their stomachs.[9] He would later claim to have found metastases to the lungs of these rats.

At the time other investigators challenged his results with experiments of their own. It was ultimately established that the lesions in the stomach were not cancerous but probably due to irritation. The lung lesions in the rats described by Fibiger could be reproduced with a diet deficient in vitamin A.

The impact of this on subsequent recognition for work in the field of cancer was profound. The demonstration of a relationship between x-ray exposure and skin cancer reported by Jean Clonet in 1908 was ignored.[10] Also included on the list of possibilities in 1926 when Fibiger was honored was the Japanese investigator Katsusaburo Yamagiwa (1863-1930). He and his colleague Koichi Ichikawa (1888-1948) in 1915 had produced skin cancer by the repeated application of coal tar to the skin of rats.[11] This other important basic research on the genesis of cancer was never recognized by a Nobel despite eight nominations between 1925 and 1938.

Perhaps the most notable failure in timely recognition was the work of Peyton Rous at the Rockefeller Institute. Rous had reported the transfer of chicken sarcomas with a cell-free infiltrate of the neoplasms (i.e. one containing virus particles).[12] It was not until he had reached the age of 87 that Rous finally mounted the podium to receive his award in 1966. He had been considered and rejected for the prize about 20 times before this moment which he shared with surgeon Charles Huggins. Huggins was honored for his use of hormonal treatment in prostatic cancer. These represented the first awards for cancer research granted by the Nobel committees after a 40 year hiatus following the Fibiger debacle.

How many other important advances in cancer research were also unheralded in Stockholm during this long dry period? One of them was unquestionably related to the introduction of chemotherapy for the treatment of malignancies when Louis. S. Goodman, Maxwell M. Wintrobe and their associates reported on the beneficial effects of nitrogen mustard on a variety of hematological neoplasms.[13] Another important advance involved the early diagnosis of cervical cancer in women with the use of the "Pap smear."George

Papanicalaou received ten nominations between 1948 and 1951 without an award.

Ironically, despite the rejection of Fibiger's belief in infection inciting cancer, in a number of other settings (including the virus in Rous's chicken sarcomas) this has been demonstrated: the hepatitis B virus in liver cancer; the Epstein-Barr virus in certain lymphomas.

It was the discovery of another infective agent, *Helicobacter pylori* that led to the 2005 Nobel award to Barry J. Marshall and Robin Warren for elucidating the role of this bacterium in gastric cancer as well as peptic ulcer and gastritis. (The roles of the papilloma virus in cervical cancer and that of the HIV virus in AIDS-related neoplasia were recognized in 2008).

Less often referred to as a mistaken judgment is that which involved the famous Russian researcher Ivan P. Pavlov (1849-1946). Although his lasting fame is based on his work on the physiology of reflexes, his Nobel Prize in 1904 was for "demonstrating the role of the brain in controlling digestion." That this was in error was revealed by Ernest H. Starling and William M. Bayliss at University College of London with their discovery of Secretin.[14]

Their demonstration that any nervous control over pancreatic secretion was mediated by this hormone (an early use of the term) was quickly acknowledged by Pavlov to his credit.[15] Starling received four unsuccessful nominations between 1913 and 1926, three of them for Secretin. Bayliss's name appeared on two of these. Committee reports on the nominations of 1913 and 1914 were obtained.[16] Despite his co-authorship on the Secretin paper Bayliss was deemed unworthy of inclusion for consideration. It turns out that although Starling was in line for the award the onset of World War I suspended such activity between 1915 and 1918. When Starling was nominated again in 1926 his discovery was deemed "too old."[17] Could his contradiction of Pavlov's earlier work also been a factor in his rejection by the Nobel committee?

Become a surgeon

The Karolinska Institute has not been particularly partial to surgeons over the last 109 years. Only nine surgeons have received the medical prize. Among these only three were actually honored for their surgical skill: Emil Kocher for his work on the thyroid gland (1909); Alexis Carrel for his contributions to vascular suturing and organ transplantation (1912); and Joseph E. Murray for kidney transplantation (1990). The accomplishments of the others were primarily in the field of physiological research.

Ironically, one major surgical innovation was credited to a neurologist rather than a surgeon. This was for the introduction of prefrontal lobotomy for the treatment of mental disease by the Portuguese physician Egas Moniz (1949). This treatment proved to be a major blunder and was soon abandoned although Moniz's reputation survives because of his introduction of cerebral angiography.

The emphasis in the Will on accomplishments achieved "in the preceding year" works against surgeons whose discoveries, perfected on the operating room table, often take decades to achieve. An outstanding surgeon like the German Ernst Sauerbruch (1875-1939) whose innovations included a technique for operating on the open chest and thus opening the whole new field of thoracic surgery, garnered 54 nominations between 1914 and 1951 without receiving the final nod. His French counterpart in prominence as a surgical pioneer, René Leriche (1879-1955), was nominated 44 times without success.

Perhaps the greatest omission among surgeons was that of Harvey Cushing (1869-1939). He was not only a great innovator but has been recognized as the founder of neurosurgery.[18] In 1932 Cushing completed his two thousandth brain tumor removal as, according to Bliss, "...the first surgeon in history who could open ...the skull of living patients with a reasonable certainty that his operations would do more good than harm." Equally notable is the operation he devised for the pain crippling affliction of trigeminal neuralgia (ganglionectomy) and his discovery of the relations of certain pituitary adenomas to the syndrome bearing his name, "Cushing's Syndrome."

Comparable to Cushing's accomplishments in the treatment of brain tumors has been the quest of Michael E. DeBakey (1908-2008)) for the treatment of aortic aneurysms. Beginning in the 1950s DeBakey's successful treatment of abdominal aneurysms with homografts and then Dacron grafts gradually progressed proximally to more difficult surgery throughout the length of the aorta.[19] His concentration on the treatment of aortic dissections as well led to cures of this almost always rapidly fatal disease. The terminology used to specify different locations of these dissections continues to bear his name. DeBakey made contributions in many other areas of cardiovascular surgery with numerous unsuccessful Nobel nominations over the years.

The second half of the twentieth century witnessed one of the greatest advances in surgical history: the surgical treatment of cardiac disease. At first it was "extracardiac surgery," that performed on vessels leading to or from the heart and primarily for the cure or relief of congenital heart disease that electrified the medical world, There was Robert E. Gross's ligation of the persistent patent ductus arteriosus (1938); relief of aortic coarctation by Clarence Crafoord (1945); and Alfred Blalock's "blue baby operation" for cyanotic congenital heart disease (1945) with their dramatic results in desperately ill infants and children. What an impressive triumvirate that would have been at the Nobel ceremonies!

In 1948, equally dramatic was the nearly simultaneous demonstration by four different surgeons working in four different surgical centers that a lesion within the heart could be operated upon directly with success. This was mitral stenosis in rheumatic heart disease. Neither Charles P. Bailey, Dwight E. Harken, Horace G. Smithy nor Russell C. Brock would receive the honor of a Nobel Prize. Coronary artery by-pass grafting as performed by René Favaloro and others for the relief of coronary artery obstructions would become at one point the most common surgical procedure performed in the United States. This major advancement for a major disease has been ignored.

Given the author's background as a cardiologist who lived through these exciting years the emphasis here has been on surgery of the heart. No doubt others with different backgrounds have their own forgotten favorites in medicine as well as surgery.

Die prematurely

Although Nobel's will stipulated that his annual prizes be awarded for work done in the preceding year it soon became obvious that this was impractical. It often happens that several years might be required to pass before the significance of a major discovery is recognized. Such a period might also be helpful in weeding out those discoveries that turn out not to fulfill their initial promise. Such delays have not often proved critical in the proper recognition of major contributions unless, of course, the potential award winner happened to die before he or she might otherwise have been honored.

As already pointed out, posthumous awards have not been allowed so that any monies granted could enable young investigators singled out to continue on with their work.

The most celebrated occurrence of a nominee dying before a prize could be realized involved Rosalind E. Franklin. It was her x-ray diffraction photographs of DNA that provided the critical clue to James D. Watson and Francis Crick in constructing their model of this critical substance.[20] Shortly after this Franklin left her position at Kings College, London for Birkbeck College to work on the tobacco mosaic and polio viruses. She developed ovarian cancer in 1956 and died in 1958 at the age of 37. Watson and Crick shared the 1962 prize with Maurice Wilkins, an associate of Franklin's at Kings with whom she had frequently crossed swords. It is generally agreed that had Franklin survived she would have merited the prize and, given the limitation of the award to a maximum of three individuals Wilkins might have been left out.

Less recognized in this context is the failure of the Nobel hierarchy to recognize the monumental achievement involved with the discovery of the household mosquito *Aëdes aegypti* as the transmitter of yellow fever. The Yellow Fever Board headed by Walter Reed and including Jesse W. Lazear, James Carroll and Aristides Agramonte proved in a series of reports between 1899 and 1900 that the Cuban physician Carlos J. Finlay had been right about the carrier of the disease some years earlier. Work on infectious diseases had been a high priority in the early years of the Nobel awards in medicine. Five of the first ten of these were for discoveries in this field and the very first two awards, those in 1901 and 1902, had been given to Emil van Behring for his work on diphtheria antitoxin and Ronald Ross for his work on the transmission of malaria. Certainly the yellow fever discovery was of equal import. Why was this accomplishment not also honored?

Perhaps the similarity of the yellow fever research to that of Manson deprived it of its uniqueness in the minds of the judges. However also possibly militating against an award for the yellow fever research was the early death of some of the principals involved. Lazear died from yellow fever in 1900 at the age of 34 while still in Cuba. Reed died from appendicitis in 1902 at the age of 51. James Carroll died in 1907 succumbing to illness at the age of 53. Finlay, however, lived until 1915; Agramonte survived until 1931; and Colonel, later General William C. Gorgas, the army officer who oversaw the practical elimination of yellow fever from Havana as well as in the Panama Canal Zone later on by instituting preventive measures, lived until 1920. In the years of consideration soon after the work had been completed the deaths of Lazear, Carroll and especially Reed may have worked to exclude their accomplishment from consideration.

You do not have to be young to die prematurely, at least in terms of reaching the goal of a Nobel Prize. The surgeon Judah Folkman (1933-2008) was an extremely original thinker who hit upon the idea that the growth of neoplasms could be angiogenesis dependent and that by attacking this element in their survival we could help desperately ill cancer patients. He had worked upon this hypothesis over 30 years at the time of his death at the age of 74 in 2008, just when increasingly promising clinical results seemed to be forthcoming.

Another case of a premature demise involved Solomon A. Berson who, for 22 years, worked closely with the physicist Roslyn Yalow in the development of radioimmunoassay. He died at the age of 53 in 1972. When she received a Nobel in 1977 she made it clear that had Berson lived he would certainly be sharing it with her. The author was told a story about Berson that could not be corroborated but is nonetheless intriguing: that he was obsessed about dying prematurely because so many of his male forbears had succumbed in this way.

Supposedly it was this premonition that drove him unceasingly toward his professional goals. To what extent may others have been driven by their sense of mortality and to what extent have such individuals been denied the pleasure of their just professional rewards by an abbreviated life span?

Become a junior partner

Some of the most unsettling controversies involving the Nobel Prize have involved the recognition, or more precisely, the non-recognition of the contributions of junior members of a research team.

In 1943 Albert Schatz (1920-2005) was a 23 year-old graduate student working under Selman A. Waksman at Rutgers University when he volunteered to search for an antibiotic for the treatment of tuberculosis. Working mostly alone in a basement where he often slept and receiving only a pittance of $40 per month, he was also at considerable risk of infection working with viable bacteria. After three and a half months he finally isolated the antibiotic streptomycin which would prove to be the first effective medical therapy for this dread disease. He was first author on the paper announcing the discovery.[21]

In 1952 it was Waksman alone who received the Nobel Prize for this discovery. For years Schatz complained about his being excluded as co-discoverer. Even before the awarding of the Nobel he had reason to complain about the distribution of royalties obtained from the mass production of the antibiotic. He had been led to forego any financial claims under the impression that all such funds would go to Rutgers for the promotion of science. He then learned that Waksman was receiving part of the royalties despite the former assurances to the contrary. In 1950 he sued Waksman and Rutgers University and in an out of court settlement won a three percent share while Waksman received ten percent. After enduring many bitter years of being considered a crank and malcontent in some quarters, Schatz received an acknowledgment of his contribution in the form of the 1994 Rutgers University Medal, the institution's highest honor.

The dispute that arose after the 1923 award for the discovery of insulin was even more heated.[22] The four principals were Frederick G. Banting, the young surgeon who spearheaded the project; Charles H. Best, the medical student who worked closely with him throughout; James B. Collip, a brilliant biochemist who joined them later and was instrumental in isolating the hormone; and J. R. Macleod, the professor of physiology at the University of Toronto, within whose department the research was conducted.

All four might easily have been included but the prize was limited to three individuals. Banting was an obvious choice. Macleod, who was a world authority on carbohydrate metabolism, was also felt to be an important contributor. But Best's name was not even included on any of the nominations, "…a circumstance that probably gave the Committee a wrong impression of Best's share in the discovery."[23] Best and Collip were both ignored. On learning of Best's exclusion Banting was furious and publicly announced his sharing of the financial prize with his youthful assistant. Macleod responded in kind by splitting his financial award with Collip. Despite their exclusion Best and Collip both went on to distinguished academic careers in Canada.

In both the streptomycin and insulin cases pre-twentieth century tradition cast a shadow. There was the assumption that any discoveries coming out of the laboratory of a distinguished professor automatically emerged under his name. In contrast to such unsettling instances of such injustice to younger colleagues there are other heart warming examples of Nobel history that can be recalled.

When the 1934 prize for "liver therapy in cases of anemia" was announced, George R. Minot and William P. Murphy were honored for their introduction of the liver diet for the successful treatment of pernicious anemia. George H. Whipple at the University of Rochester was added because of his long history of research on diet in the treatment of anemia, notably iron deficiency anemia induced in dogs. Dr. Frieda Robscheit-Robbins had worked with Whipple as a co-investigator for 30 years and had been co-author or first author on a number of important papers published. Although she was overlooked by the Nobel committee, Whipple, in recognition of her contributions, shared a good portion of the monetary award with her and with other faithful laboratory workers under him.

When a Nobel representative visited the laboratory of John F. Enders in connection with a future prize for his laboratory's achievement in tissue culture techniques for the poliomyelitis virus Enders made it clear that any award would have to include his two junior collaborators, Thomas H. Weller and Frederick C. Robbins.[24] All three shared the prize in 1954.

Enders' graciousness toward his co-workers was admirable. One wonders, however, how many more worthy young investigators in similar positions to that of Weller and Robbins might have been overlooked. Occasionally history provides a hint at such hidden treasures.

In 1960 Peter Medawar at the University of London shared the prize with Frank Macfarlane Burnet of Australia for their contributions to the understanding of acquired immunological tolerance. Following the award, in a letter to the wife of his associate Leslie B. Brent he wrote, regarding the latter, "And anyway it was his PhD thesis, not mine, that won the prize… and I do so wish he could have shared the titular award." The letter was not made public until almost fifty years later when it was reproduced in a memoir of Brent's entitled *Sunday's Child?*[25] It is likely that had Medawar been made aware of the approaching prize he would have enthusiastically endorsed Brent's inclusion in the honor. To his credit, Brent never harbored any bitterness toward Medawar because of having been overlooked. If the Nobel investigators had done their work a bit more thoroughly this would have, undoubtedly, not been the case.

How many more similar stories might be told? Given the nature of such deficiencies in the system attempting to estimate the number of these is beyond conjecture.

Defy the rule of three

According to Article 4 of the Nobel statutes "in no case may a prize be divided between more than three persons." What is the rationale for this? It certainly was not stipulated in the will. Is it because extending it beyond three people would result in too small a financial reward to relieve any economic hardships for the recipient(s)? The penury of Pierre and Marie Curie who shared the 1903 Physics Prize with Henri Becquerel is part of the treasured Nobel lore. They lived in a sixth floor garret where they had to sleep fully clothed in winter to protect themselves from the cold. Their work place was no better: glass paneled, damp and also unheated. They certainly needed the financial windfall that the prize carried with it. Today, however, especially with the frequently long time interval between discovery and prize, the recipients are more likely to be middle-aged, gainfully employed and in possession of substantial research grants from government or private sources. So money does not explain the rule.

Is there fear of diminishing the prestige of the prize by spreading it too thin among too many people? With 6.5 billion souls on earth, increasing the number from three to four or five would not represent much of a dilution factor. With the increasing complexity of research it often takes more than one or two individuals or even three to reach a desired goal. Certainly life might have been simpler and less painful all around if all four of the insulin researchers had been included. And had Rosalind Franklin lived to 1962 it would not have been necessary to agonize over eliminating Maurice Wilkins while sustaining the nominations of Franklin, Watson and Crick.

The 1988 prize for discoveries elucidating the effects of nitric oxide on the cardiovascular system went to Robert F. Furchgott, Louis J. Ignarro and Ferid Murad. Omitted here was the name of Salvatore Moncada who, among an impressive number of papers on the subject, had the most cited paper in the literature. Many scientists bristled at the failure to honor Moncada, including Furchgott.[26]

There are probably many other instances of this error of omission unknown to the author. It is worthy of note that the same article of the Foundation limiting the award to three individuals allows for the committee involved to award an institution or association when it deems fit. The Nobel Peace Prize has often been awarded in this way (e.g The Red Cross, UNICEF, Doctors Without Borders) but not the Physiology/Medicine prize.

Become an inventor

Note in Nobel's will that in regard to the prize in physics the term "invention" is included along with "discovery," but not in reference to the award in Physiology or Medicine. This may reflect the general view at the turn of the last century that medical discoveries were made in the clinic or in laboratories filled with test tubes, burettes, pipettes and Petri dishes along with other paraphernalia associated with medical research. Machines, as such, were not looked upon as within this province.

The very first physics prize in 1901 went to Wilhelm Röentgen for the discovery of x-rays. Later ones went to other inventions such as the wireless radio, x-ray spectrometry, electron microscopy and the cloud chamber. As for medicine, early on it was not realized how great a role technology would come to play in the diagnosis and treatment of human disease. There were, however, notable exceptions to this. In 1924 Willem Einthoven was honored for his work in electrocardiography; in 1979 Allan McCormack and Godfrey Hounsfield won for developing computer assisted tomography (CT scanning); and in 2003 Paul C. Lauterbur and Peter Mansfield shared the prize for magnetic resonance imaging (MRI).

This having been noted, there remain a number of critical inventions that have led to major progress in the diagnosis and treatment of human disease but have been rejected in the deliberations of the Nobel committees for Physiology or Medicine. One candidate for this category was the invention of the electroencephalograph (EEG) by Hans Berger (1873-1941), a German physiologist cum neurologist and psychiatrist. His work on the EEG began in the 1920s but its importance not recognized until 1937 when he was accorded international acclaim for this accomplishment. There was only a short window of opportunity for the Nobel judges to honor Berger. He received six nominations between 1940 and 1950, most of them moot since, as a result of Nazi oppression, he was driven to suicide in 1941.

Among other notable absences on the Nobel roster is Willem J. Kolff (1911-2009), a Dutch physician who was the first to develop a practical artificial kidney. Amazingly this work was done while Holland was under Nazi occupation with his first success in Europe coming in 1945. This led to a visit to the United States in 1947 with more successes accumulating thereafter. Added to his work on renal failure are his contributions to the development of the heart lung machine with his work on the membrane oxygenator and the artificial heart. Most informed medical scientists are agreed about his having merited a Nobel for his work in the development of artificial organs.

A cardiologist could easily point to a number of other important inventions in his field that were deserving of notice and did not meet with the necessary approval. The heart-lung machine, first used successfully in 1953 by its inventor John H. Gibbon (1904-1973) has become an integral component to the great majority of operations being performed on the heart over the last 50 years. In Sweden physicist Carl Hellmuth Hertz (1920-1990) and physician Inge Edler (1911-2001) combined their talents to found the field of echocardiography, a boon to those wishing to perform diagnostic examinations of the heart without risk or pain. In the 1980s Michel Mirowski (1924-1990) developed the automatic implantable defibrillator, which has enabled thousands of patients to survive sudden cardiac arrest.

Even when recognizing such an important invention as MRI, it appears the Nobel committee has managed, in the view of many, to stumble. In 2003, when the medical prize was awarded to Lauterbur and Mansfield, the important pioneering work of Raymond V. Damadian was ignored. Damadian's efforts in the early 1970s preceded the work of the others and he produced the first human body scan in 1977. He was also awarded patents in 1974 for his inventions. Following the Nobel oversight Damadian took out full-page advertisements in the New York Times staking his claim.[27] Although these smacked of sensationalism, reflecting Damadian's great frustration, on careful reading of these and cooler assessments from other sources, Damadian's outrage seems justified. Nevertheless, by the rules of the Nobel Foundation, all judgments are final. Although Damadian, who left academia in 1978 to found Fonar, a commercial enterprise, has become a wealthy man, living well for one so slighted may not in the end prove to be the best revenge.

Repeat a performance

In 1912 Alexis Carrel received the prize "in recognition for his work on vascular suture and the transplantation of blood vessels and organs." Michael DeBakey may not have been in the same mold; he never did any transplantation work. However his work on the treatment of aortic aneurysms (see above) revolutionized the field and his other accomplishments in cardiovascular research should have lent sufficient weight of merit to his numerous unsuccessful nominations. Did the committees involved simply think of DeBakey's contributions as "more of the same?"

While Joseph E. Murray and E. Donnall Thomas received the prize in 1990 for kidney and bone marrow transplantation respectively, no award has ever been made for liver, heart or lung transplantation, discoveries of equal magnitude one might argue.

Become controversial

The Nobel judges have seemed ambivalent when confronted with controversy. At times they seem to have shied away from otherwise promising candidates at odds with one another; on other occasions rivals have been brought together to share in the award in Stockholm.

The poliomyelitis dispute between Albert B. Sabin and Jonas Salk over selection of a vaccine with live attenuated virus orally administered (Sabin) or a killed virus in an injectible form (Salk) was so bitter that it might be wondered if the two could be ever coaxed into the same room no less on to the same stage.[28] Although each vaccine formulation has its particular merits and both have been incorporated into modern vaccination regimens it was many years before a consensus could be reached on a health care measure that had such a profound effect in reducing the incidence of polio among populations where they were employed.

The competition over the discovery of the AIDS virus (human immunodeficiency virus or HIV) that arose between the American Robert Gallo of the National Cancer Center and the Frenchman Luc Montagnier of the Pasteur Institute has been called "The AIDS War."[29] Ultimately both groups shared in the royalties arising from the blood test that became available, but there was no sharing of a Nobel in 2008 when Gallo was excluded from this honor.

Despite examples of self-defeating competition other rivalries in the course of medical discovery have not impeded the path to a Nobel. Santiago Ramon y Cajàl, a Spanish physician, and his Italian opponent Camillo Golgi held markedly different views on the functional anatomy of the nerve fibers within the brain. The dispute went on for years, but it did not prevent a Nobel Prize from being awarded to both of them in 1906 "in recognition of their work on the structure of the nervous system."[30]

The animus between Roger Guilleman and Andrew V. Schally was perhaps even more intense owing to the fact that it was personal in many respects and lasted for over 21 years.[31] They both sought to isolate the chemicals arising at the base of the brain controlling pituitary hormone secretion. The arduous task of finding these substances, which exist in only the minutest quantities, required a back-breaking effort well worthy of the Nobel they received in 1977 "for their discoveries of the peptide hormone production of the brain."

Factors other than rivalry with another researcher have probably resulted in the denial of the award to some otherwise outstanding individuals. One possible candidate for this kind of adverse scrutiny might have been the British physiologist Ernest Starling (1866-1927) whose discovery of Secretin has already been mentioned. During his long career he was responsible for at least two other major discoveries which might have merited a Nobel prize.[32] One involved his work on lymph and capillaries determining the forces shifting fluid between the small blood vessels and the surrounding tissue space (Starling's Hypothesis). Finally there was his work on the control of cardiac function culminating in Starling's Law of the Heart which, to this day, underlies much of our understanding of normal cardiac function as well as cardiac pathophysiology.

Why was Starling denied the trappings of such success even in Great Britain where he was never knighted for his work and denied choice academic appointments? Perhaps this could be accounted for by his prickly personality. Starling was outspoken, short-tempered, impolitic and highly critical of the British system of medical education as he found it in his time. He certainly did not endear himself to the establishment. As already mentioned, he received four nominations for a Nobel, mainly for Secretin, but all were unsuccessful.

Another potential laureate was Robert A. Good (1922-2003) who had made a number of fundamental contributions to immunology. However his reputation was irrevocably stained by his association with William Summerlin. It was Summerlin who, while working under Good at the Sloan-Kettering Institute in New York, actually painted white mice black when he could not repeat the skin transplantation experiment he had previously performed at the University of Minnesota.

Sigmund Freud (1856-1938) received a total of 32 nominations between 1915 and 1938. Toward the end of his life, if for no other reason than the financial aspects of the reward, it would have been very welcome. The Nazis had stripped him of his assets before he was allowed to leave Vienna and at the end of his life he and his family were living in very straitened circumstances.[33] Always the realist, however, Freud knew that the decision makers were against him and that he would never outlive their hostility. Another possible factor in the late thirties was that a militant Germany was in the ascendancy and some of the Swedish judges may not have wished to offend their bellicose neighbor by selecting Freud.

Ride the crest of a distant wave

Medical research, like many other scientific, artistic or other cultural endeavors, has its changing trends.[34] During the earliest decades of the Nobel awards the prizes prominently honored work in infectious diseases and immunology (six of the first thirteen between 1901 and 1913). Research in digestion, hormones, neurobiology, cancer and other medical areas of interest have had, over the years, a more modest representation. Recently, however, it has been the fields of genetics and molecular biology that have dominated the awards. The prize given in 1958 to George Beadle, Edward Tatum and Joshua Lederberg for their contributions to the field of genetics might be looked upon as the start of this trend. Between 1958 and 2007 19 prizes, almost half of all awarded, were given for discoveries in these rapidly emerging fields. As a result of this new focus in modern medical research even fairly extraordinary accomplishments in other areas (e.g. nutrition, chemotherapy, intermediary metabolism, surgery, circulatory physiology) may not have received their full due. Medical researchers whose careers are tied to these other currently less fashionable fields may discover that interest in their kind of research has cooled. They have crested on a wave of medical research that has already passed from view in the sea of scientific discovery.

Possess the wrong pedigree

Although usually used in reference to bloodlines in animal husbandry, the term "pedigree" might also loosely be used to describe the racial, ethnic, cultural, religious, educational and even financial backgrounds of individuals as well as gender. The presence of so many white males, usually of European background, on either side of the Atlantic Ocean as predominant among Nobel laureates is understandable. After all, like favors like when it comes to such considerations even when such a biased selection is unconsciously made. The paucity of women, with only seven receiving this honor in physiology or medicine over the century of the awards is not surprising.

Alfred Nobel reflected an internationalist's view of all this when he concluded in his will that "…the most worthy shall receive the prize, whether he be Scandinavian or not." How well has this wish been borne out over the years?

The Japanese, who have a notable history of accomplishments in medical research, have not fared too well in the selection process, at least as it has pertained to the Prize in Physiology or Medicine. Susumi Tonegawa, who received the prize in 1987 "for his discovery of the genetic principle for generation of antibody diversity," is the sole exception. It should be noted, however, that although he was born in Japan and received his undergraduate degree in chemistry there, much of his training and research took place in the United States and Switzerland.

In the early years of the twentieth century young ambitious Japanese came to the West to attach themselves to prominent figures in laboratory medicine. Sakashiro Hata, who joined Paul Ehrlich in March of 1909 may be looked upon as more a victim of poor timing than anything else. He did much of the work resulting later that year in the discovery of compound 606 (Salvarsan), the first really effective treatment for syphilis. Unfortunately for him, just a short time before in 1906 Ehrlich had received a Nobel along with Elie Metchnikoff for "their work on the theory of immunity." If Ehrlich had not been so recently honored he may well have shared the prize for Salvarsan with Hata.

Earlier Shibasakuro Kitasato had an even better chance at the prize. A pupil of Koch, he had already discovered the tetanus bacillus. He then joined von Behring at the Koch Institute in 1899 as a collaborator in the work on antitoxins. The very first Nobel Prize in Physiology or Medicine was awarded to von Behring for his work on serum therapy in 1901. He was not joined by Kitasato. The overlooking of Yamagiwa and Ichikawa, who did their work in Japan on skin cancer induction by irritants has already been mentioned. Hideyo Noguchi (1876-1928), among many other accomplishments in infectious disease, demonstrated the spirochete, *Treponema pallidum* as the cause of syphilis of the brain. Despite a number of nominations he never received the Nobel prize for any of this important work.

Salvador Moncada, a native Honduran, might also represent a victim of some form of xenophobia. His failure to be included in the award for the work on nitric oxide has already been noted. In later years, commenting on his placement within the research establishment he replied, "That [a high position] would be difficult for a Latin American Jew who didn't go to the right schools or universities, comes from an almost unknown country and speaks English with the wrong accent."[35]

Jews have historically been systematically excluded from medical education in Europe and even the United States until relatively recently. Scientific research in Great Britain was traditionally the preserve of the wealthy gentry for much of its history. In this country academic medical pursuits were predominantly dominated by WASPS (white Anglo-Saxon protestants), especially those financially independent and emerging from the top tier American universities. Despite this, as attested by Nobel laureate Arthur Kornberg to a colleague not long ago, New York's egalitarian free public school, City College, could account for 24 Nobel laureates (all categories), 23 of them Jewish.[36] And a number of other Jews in Medicine or Physiology from Ehrlich on could be added to this roster. In this respect, the performance of the Nobel Foundation has been exemplary.

Be humble

In the sciences as well as in business, government and the arts there have always been the "ins" and the "outs." Members of the "in" group are likely to be adept at the social graces. They attend the right meetings, shake the right hands, pat the right backs, boost the right egos and get themselves appointed to the right committees. Oswald Avery (1877-1955) was the complete antithesis of this. One of his collaborators at the Rockefeller Institute years later would describe him as "…a small man who was quite restrained."[37] A lifelong bachelor, Avery led a secluded personal existence. He hated to talk in public and even when he had to give a presidential address before the Society of American Bacteriologists he refused to have it published. He may have suffered from depression as well and later developed a marked tremor possibly related to thyroid disease. The paper he published in 1944 with Colin McLeod and Maclyn McCarty showing that deoxyribonucleic acid (DNA) contains the factors of heredity established a blueprint for much of what was to come in the field of molecular biology.[38]

Avery had already received 17 nominations in the years preceding this for other contributions to his field; between 1946 and 1951 there were 16 additional nominations for the DNA work. In a rare disclosure of reasons underlying the decisions of the Nobel committees it was claimed that this discovery was not fully accepted until 1952.[39] Could Avery's reticence about his own accomplishments have been an additional factor during his lifetime?

Charles Weissmann may represent a similar case of an inability at self-promotion .[40] It was Stanley Prusiner who won the prize in 1977 for his discovery of prions, a new biological element of infection. It has been shown to account for scrapie in sheep, mad cow disease and a similar disease of the brain in humans (Creutzfeldt-Jakob disease). This was an exciting breakthrough to which Weissmann contributed significantly by discovering the structure of the protein involved. Unlike Prusiner, who, it is believed, actively pursued the prize, Weissmann engaged in no similar efforts and was not included in the honor.

How many other worthy scientists might fit into this category of the overlooked? Given the nature of the personality characteristics involved – modesty and or reserve – they may be difficult to detect even by those interested in uncovering them.

Stop an epidemic

The army officer William C. Gorgas (1844-1920), following up on the yellow fever findings of Walter Reed and his associates, headed the drive to practically wipe out this and other insect borne diseases from Havana, Cuba. Similar efforts by him later on in Panama enabled the completion of the Panama Canal.

Donald Henderson (b.1928), as head of the World Health Organization Global Smallpox Eradication Campaign achieved the complete eradication of this horrible disease by a worldwide vaccination campaign with the last reported case occurring in 1977.

Norman E. Borlaug (1914-2009), through his development of improved strains of wheat became known as "The Father of the Green Revolution" which stemmed the tide of starvation in many parts of the world.

After implementation of his polio vaccine program in 1954 Jonas Salk oversaw the reduction of this disease in the United States from 25 per 100,000 in 1953 to .5 per 100,000 between 1954 and 1961. Albert Sabin had a similar success with his oral vaccine in the Soviet Union.

None of these scientists received the Nobel Prize in Physiology or Medicine although Borlaug did receive a Peace Prize in 1970. As pointed out in a recent Lancet editorial, there is nothing restricting from consideration such epidemiological accomplishments.[41] This is clearly stated in Article 4 of the Statutes. Nevertheless the members of the Nobel selection committees have acted otherwise. It is revealing that while Salk and Sabin were rejected for work that has saved many thousands of lives and prevented unknown millions of crippling after effects, the award for poliomyelitis went to John Enders and his assistants for developing a method of culturing the virus. Obviously it is the figure of the isolated scientist, working late into many nights before achieving the Eureka moment that has captured the imagination of these judges rather than that of the public health crusaders who have successfully labored to save countless lives among the peoples of the world.

CONCLUSIONS

Since the passing of Albert Nobel the world of medical research has grown enormously. During his lifetime there were a few notable research institutes producing excellent results in Europe, but Nobel realized how inadequate they were to the worldwide need for medical and other scientific advances.. They were also inadequate to the need for the training of future investigators for the benefit of mankind. Today, especially with the burgeoning of powerful government sponsors such as the National Institutes of Health and the National Science Foundation in this country, similar research establishments in Europe and the World Health Organization, funding for such research has become infinitely greater. These have been supplemented by the growth of many private foundations, probably at least one dedicated to every major human ailment identifiable. It is unlikely that even if the Nobel Foundation ceased to exist that this would represent a significant impediment to future medical research.

What then is the role of the Nobel Prizes in this rapidly changing world? After all is said and done and all the inconsistencies and possible flaws have been revealed it turns out that, to a large extent, the Nobel awards continue to adhere to their benefactor's original purpose: the appreciation and propagation of leading edge medical research.

And "leading edge" it is indeed. In the accompanying table are listed some of the discoveries for which physiology/medical prizes have been awarded in recent years (Table 11.1). This is a time during which we have experienced what Renée Fox has called "the molecularization of medicine." It is unlikely that many physicians, no less lay persons, have the faintest idea of what they may mean. But that is just the point. Each generation of the past has faced the same challenge as the new medicine of the time begins to take hold.

Table 11.1. Recent Physiology or Medicine Nobel Awards

Year	For the discovery of:
1983	mobile genetic elements.
1989	cellular origin of retroviral oncogenes.
1994	G-proteins and their role in signal transduction in cells.
1999	proteins that have intrinsic signals that govern their transport and localization in the cell.
2006	RNA interference-gene silencing by double-stranded RNA.
2007	principles for introducing specific gene modifications in mice by use of embryonic stem cells.

Medical progress will go on whatever the various trappings of success offered by a grateful society. Very few medical scientists actually plan to win the great prize. The way it really happens most of the time was well expressed by Nobel laureate J. Michael Bishop who, tongue in cheek, entitled his memoir *How to Win a Nobel Prize:*

> *The title of the book notwithstanding, I have an aversion to using the word "win" when speaking of the Nobel Prize. The verb inspires a competitive view of science that I find repugnant. Harold Varmus*

and I ran no race. We did our work and it happened to lead to an amazing place. There was no talk of a Nobel Prize when we began our experiments and none when we had our discovery in hand – the full significance of the discovery was not immediately apparent.[42]

All true medical scientists are motivated primarily by an irresistible need to understand the functioning of the human organism and the need to determine the causes of and treatments for the diseases that might afflict it. And they will continue to do so – with or without a Nobel at the end of the road.

ACKNOWLEDGMENT: Professor Istvàn Hargittai kindly reviewed an early draft of this manuscript.

REFERENCES

1. Sohlman R, Schück H. *Nobel. Dynamite and Peace.* New York: Cosmopolitan Book Corp., 1929; Mayer EP. *Dynamite and Peace. The Story of Alfred Nobel.* Boston: Little Brown, 1958; Fant K. *Alfred Nobel. A Biography.* New York: Arcade Publishing, 1991; Feldman B. *The Nobel Prize. A History of Genius, Controversy and Prestige.* New York: Arcade Publishing, 2000.

2. Schück H, Sohlman R, Österling A, Liljestrand G, Westgren A, Siegban M, Schou A, Stahl NK. *Nobel. The Man and His Prizes.* Norman: University of Oklahoma Press, 1951. (reprinted).

3. Schück H, Sohlman R et al. *Nobel. The Man and His Prizes.* 2nd *Edition.* New York: Elsevier, 1962; Odelberg W, Ed. *Nobel. The Man and His Prizes.* 3rd *Edition.* New York: Elsevier, 1972.

4. Nobel Foundation, Statutes *of the Nobel Foundation.* Stockholm: Nobel Foundation, 2005.

5. Details and clarifications furnished by Prof. Ann-Margreth Jörnvall, Administrator, the Nobel Committee for Physiology or Medicine, Karolinska Institutet, May 2008 – February 2009.

6. Lindsten J, Ringertz N in Levinovitz AW and Ringertz N. *The Nobel Prize. The First 100 Years.* London: Imperial College Press, 2001, 115-116.

7. Zuckerman H. *Scientific Elite. Nobel Laureates in the United States.* New Brunswick: Transaction Publishers, 1996; Raju TNK. *The Nobel Chronicles. A Handbook of Nobel Prizes in Physiology or Medicine 1901-2000.* Chicago: T.N.K. Raju, 2002; Hargittai I. *The Road to Stockholm. Nobel Prizes, Science and Scientists.* Oxford: Oxford University Press, 2002; Bishop JM. *How to Win the Nobel Prize.* Cambridge: Harvard University Press, 2003.

8. Odelberg, *Nobel,* 141-278.

9. Fibiger J. "Recherches sur un nematode et sur sa faculté de provoquer des néoformations papillomateuses dans l'estomac du rat," *Acad. Royale Sci Lettres Danemark,* 1913, 1-41.

10. Mustacchi P, Shimkin MB. Radiation Cancer and Jean Clunet. *Cancer,* 1956; 9: 1073-1074.

11. Yamagiwa K, Ichikawa KJ. Experimental study of the pathogenesis of carcinoma. *J Cancer Research,* 1918; 3: 1-29.

12. Rous P. A sarcoma of the fowl transmissible by an agent separable from the tumor cells. *J Exp. Med* 1911;13: 397-411.

13. Goodman LS, Wintrobe MM, Dameshek W et al. Nitrogen mustard therapy. *J Am Med Assoc* 1946;132:126-132.

14. Bayliss WM , Starling EH. On the causation of the so called "peripheral reflex secretion" of the pancreas (Preliminary communication). *Proc Royal Soc B* 1902;69:352-353.

15. Henderson J. *A Life of Ernest Starling.* Oxford: Oxford University Press, 2005, 58.

16. Courtesy of A-M Jörnvall. Translation by Kristine Antoniades, M.D.

17. Liljestrand G in Shück and Sohlman, *Nobel, 2*nd *Edition,* 225-226.

18. Bliss M. *Harvey Cushing. A Life in Surgery.* Oxford: Oxford University Press, 2005.

19. DeBakey ME. The development of vascular surgery. *Am J Surg* 1979;137:697-738.

20. Watson JD, Crick FH. Molecular structure of nucleic acids. *Nature* 1953;171: 737-738.

21. Schatz A, Bugie E, Waksman SA. Streptomycin, a substance exhibiting antibiotic activity against gram positive and gram negative bacteria. *Proc Soc Exp Biol Med* 1944;57:244-248.

22. Bliss M. *The Discovery of Insulin.* Chicago: University of Chicago Press, 1982.

23. Liljestrand G in *Nobel, 1*st *Edition,* 1952, 223.

24. Robbins FC, in Hargittai I. *Candid Science III. Conversations with Famous Biomedical Scientists.* London: Imperial College Press, 2002, 503.

25. Brent LB. *Sunday's Child? A Memoir.* United Kingdom: Bank House Books, 2009.

26. Furchgott RF in Hargittai, *Candid Science II,* 593.

27. New York Times 2003: "Visual proof that this shameful wrong must be righted (Nov. 11, F3); "The year's Nobel Prize in Medicine (Dec. 9, A16-17.)

28. Weisse AB, *Medical Odysseys. The Different and Sometimes Unexpected Pathways to Twentieth Century Medical Discoveries.* New Brunswick: Rutgers University Press, 1991, 158-185.

29. Hellman H. *Great Feuds in Medicine.* New York: Wiley and Sons, 2001, 165-183.

30. Ibid., 91-104.

31. Wade N. Guillemin and Schally: A race spurred by rivalry. *Science* 1978;200: 510-513.

32. Henderson, *A Life of Starling.*

33. Jones E. *The Life and Work of Sigmund Freud. Vol 3.* New York: Basic Books, 1957.

34. Levinovitz AW, Ringertz N. *The Nobel Prize. The First 100 Years.* London: Imperial College Press, 2001.

35. Moncada S in Hargittai, *Candid Science II,* 576.

36. Levi-Montalcini R in Hargittai, *Candid Science II,* 369.

37. McCarty M in Hargittai, *Candid Science II,* 29.

38. Avery OT, McLeod CM, McCarty M. Studies of the chemical nature of the substance inducing transformation of pneumococcal types. *J Exp Med* 1944; 79:137-158.

39. Liljestrand G, Bernhard CG in Odelberg, *Nobel 3rd Edition,* 201.

40. Hargittai, *Candid Science II,* 460, 467-497.

41. Editorial. Narrowness of Nobel Awards for Physiology or Medicine. *The Lancet* 1999;354:1399.

42. Bishop JM. *How to Win the Nobel Prize.* Cambridge: Harvard University Press, 2003, 33.

12

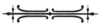

DREAMWORK

I LIVE TWO SEPARATE LIVES. The first is that of an aging cardiologist and medical historian. The other takes over each night as I fall asleep and enter a dream world of infinite variety and emotional involvement. There is not a night's slumber from which I emerge without the memory of some fascinating dream or two with which to bombard my wife at the breakfast table. This she has good-naturedly tolerated for over forty years. Close friends and colleagues have also been the kindly recipients of my nocturnal adventures when I have managed to recall the details into the following days.

The dreams are not all pleasant. Fifty years out of medical school and I am still experiencing variations of a recurring anxiety dream concerning failure at examinations. I cannot locate the examination room; I arrive too late to pick up the test forms; pencils break and pens run dry; I cannot find a seat with adequate lighting to enable me to read the questions which, oftentimes, are printed in type too small to be read; the examination papers become jumbled or fall from my hands; I spend so much time on the first few questions that at the time of the closing bell I have yet to even glance at the bulk of the remaining questions. In various combinations and of varying severity such imagined mishaps combine to awaken me in a fearful sweat all too often.

There are compensations to such unpleasant experiences as this. Interestingly enough for a physician, I have never appeared physically ill in any of my dreams. Then there are the occasional erotic episodes to be enjoyed and kept to oneself. Notably there is one treasured recurring dream of wish fulfillment. Throughout my life I have never hidden the fact that my real life's ambition was to have become a leading operatic tenor. My lasting regret is that I never "gave it a shot" despite the unlikelihood of success in such a highly competitive field. Growing up during The Great Depression with parents who were economically ravaged by it, I was encouraged to enter a more reliable field of endeavor. Medicine, the law and accountancy were particularly favored for ambitious young men of my generation and I finally opted for the first of these. Although I achieved some measure of success as an academic cardiologist there has always remained the nagging thought of what might have been.

In my dream world I suffer no such impediments to vocal ambition. I find myself backstage at an opera house much like the Metropolitan in New York if not that venerable institution itself. In a nod to reality I am no longer a youngster but someone advancing in age to a point at which my voice may have passed its peak. For years the management has made unfulfilled promises to give me a chance at performing in public and it is beginning to seem that they never will. Then, at a critical moment the leading tenor is suddenly incapacitated on stage and I, the backup, am called upon to fill in. The opera is always Puccini and the aria I deliver is always one of his finest, something like "Nessun dorma" from *Turandot*. Naturally I bring the house down despite the fact that I do not speak Italian and have to fake the words during my time on stage. No matter; it is the melody that I firmly command and that conquers all.

Other recurring themes or elements in my dreams are not so easily explained. Why, for instance, do I frequently appear barefooted? This mystery went unsolved for years until recently when my subconscious came to the rescue. In this particular variation of the theme I am a student at a prestigious Ivy League university and am returning some books to the library. I am adequately attired with the exception of footwear, a deficiency noted by a distinguished senior professor who is present and observing me. In as calm a manner as he can manage he inquires as to why I am making a spectacle of myself in this way. With equal *sang froid* I enlighten him with an explanation. I have a habit of frequently losing footwear and when I lose a slipper or shoe I believe I would look even more ridiculous wearing only one slipper rather than none at all. The scene suddenly changes to the next day and the kindly professor is again present during my arrival at the book return desk. Triumphantly he presents me with a box in which I find a complete pair of new slippers. I hasten to inform him that it might be premature for him to rejoice in his solution to the problem for, in all likelihood, I would soon be losing one of the new pair of slippers and be traipsing around the campus once again completely barefooted.

Of course there is undoubtedly something more darkly Freudian going on concerning the case of the naked feet but I am in no great hurry to find out what. I take the view of the once popular humorist Harry Golden who stated that he was already conscious of so many psychological problems with which he had to contend that the last thing he needed was a psychiatrist to pile a few more on his plate.

I have been told that people who have intense dream lives tend to be very creative. Graham Greene's psychiatrist had him keep a notepad at his bedside and record his dreams as soon as he awoke. Some of these are believed to have wound up in his novels. Although I do not claim to have the creative powers of a legendary literary figure like Greene I suppose it might do me some good to follow suit. Unfortunately I have never had either the discipline or sufficient motivation to do so. I can recall only two occasions when I was routed out of my bed by a dream and managed to write it down. One of these dreams, a long and detailed one, actually was a complete short story that I later included in a collection of writings I had published. The other was the foot story I have just related and also wanted to share with others.

All this calls to mind the lyrics of a popular song of long ago: *When I grow too old to dream I'll have you to remember."* As the years roll on I am sure that there will be much to remember, but I doubt that I will ever grow too old to dream.

13

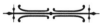

THE UMDNJ DEBACLE:
A SCANDAL IN ACADEMIA

THE UNIVERSITY OF MEDICINE and Dentistry of New Jersey is purported to be the largest free standing institution of its kind within the United States. It therefore was of considerable concern to learn that early in 2005 a remarkable series of investigative reports about disturbing irregularities at the health care giant began to appear in the Newark Star-Ledger. Among other items, these included:

- The awarding of 495.5 million dollars in no-bid contracts between 2002 and 2005.
- Possible over billing Medicare and Medicaid by University Hospital in the tens of millions of dollars.
- An award of $75,000 dollars to an associate of former Governor McGreevey for consultative work that apparently had not been performed.
- A total of $83,700 paid for chauffeuring of a Board of Concerned Citizens member back and forth from her home in the Poconos to Newark.
- Conflict of interests of a number of trustees questioning the ethics of their appointments.
- The hiring of State Senator Wayne Bryant at a no-show job paying $35,000 a year by the dean of the School of Osteopathic Medicine, R. Michael Gallagher, in return for diverting funds from the state to his school.

Such were the number and severity of possibly illegal and/or unethical acts that a former Federal Judge, Herbert Stein, was put in place to monitor the institution. This did not end until December 31, 2007.

To many of us who had been on the scene for much of that institution's history this came as no great surprise. From the time of its birth as the Seton Hall College of Medicine and Dentistry to its present status as a health care behemoth, UMDNJ has been embroiled in politics and controversy. It was political maneuvering that finally enabled the Catholic Church to preside over what were to be the first successful medical and dental schools in the state. It was politics that located them in Jersey City.

Hudson County has had a long history of corruption and Jersey City was the quintessential example of such doings during the time when Frank Hague was mayor (1917-1947). It was he who, when once questioned about the legality of one of his actions, famously replied "I am the law." But there was another side to Boss Hague and pertinent to the present discussion. He was determined to bring first rate health care to all the citizens of his community and he built the Jersey City Medical Center and the Margaret Hague Maternity Hospital to accomplish this goal. As a result of such munificence he was called by at least one observer, a medical pioneer of the time, Dr. Lena Edwards, "the good thief."

Hague was succeeded as power broker by one time subordinate John V. Kenny, who actually ran as a reform candidate but, once elected, proved even more rapacious than his predecessor. Although he was mayor only from 1949 to 1953 he remained in control as head of the Democratic Hudson County machine through various mayoral puppets until he was indicted in 1971 and convicted of conspiracy and extortion.

The activities of this political cabal were in full swing when I first arrived as an instructor in medicine at the then Seton Hall College of Medicine in Jersey City in 1963 having just completed specialty training in cardiovascular disease at the University of Utah. I became part of the department of medicine's cardiology division which was actually located in the B.S. Pollak Hospital for Chest Diseases, a county facility unlike the city-owned Jersey City Medical Center and the Margaret Hague. We constituted the Thomas J. White Institute, named after a prominent local cardiologist whom we never saw and who never referred a single patient to our top notch laboratory while I was there. What I remember most about this period, aside from the exciting intellectual atmosphere at the school that had only been started in 1954, was the political climate in which we operated. Administrative staff were mostly political appointees with questionable qualifications and every Friday afternoon, our chief of cardiology, Dr. Harper K. Hellems, was required to vacate his rather plush office in order to allow a congregation of future felons to gather there and, we believed, split up the weekly pie – and it was not pizza.

The Archdiocese of Newark, which had originally underwritten the school, began to realize that this was beyond its financial capabilities. By 1965 the school was already seven million dollars in debt and in order to keep both the medical and dental schools viable, the state of New Jersey took them over at this time. At this point the Jersey City Mayor, Thomas Whelan, attempted to seize an opportunity to unload the financially failing Jersey City Medical Center on the state as well. When he was refused Whelan issued an expulsion order depriving the school of the vital teaching beds at the Medical Center for house staff and students during their clinical years.

A special committee of experts on medical education was invited to advise the new state school, The New Jersey College of Medicine and Dentistry, of the necessary land and facilities that would be required for new construction at a yet to be determined site. They indicated that about 100 to 150 acres would be required for this purpose. The recently available 138 acre Dodge Estate in Madison filled the bill perfectly in the eyes of most of the faculty and a clear majority of us actually voted in favor of this. However, before this could occur, the mayor of Newark, Hugh Addonizio, intent on getting the school for his own city, blithely offered 185 acres in Newark for the project, a land grant that was completely beyond his power to deliver. Despite the obviously fraudulent nature of the Newark offer, the trustees turned down Madison and, probably pressured by Lyndon Johnson's administration, elected Newark as our final destination. So we wound up in 1968 in Newark with only 56 acres. Not too long afterward Addonizio wound up in jail.

The site in Newark was in the Central Ward adjacent to the old Newark City Hospital – renamed Martland Hospital after a famous Essex county medical examiner, Harrison Martland. The housing that would have to be cleared in the process contained predominantly African-Americans and included many private homes of good quality that were highly treasured by the occupants. The resulting displacement of these families probably helped to ignite the 1967 riots which demolished large sections of real estate throughout the city and from which Newark, to this day, has failed to recover completely.

This was the atmosphere greeting the first President of the New Jersey College of Medicine and Dentistry, Dr. Robert R. Cadmus (1966-1971) and his successor, Dr. Stanley S. Bergen, Jr. who presided over the institution for the next 27 years until 1998 and who, largely, may be held accountable for its successes as well as some of its failures. In 1981 the institution became designated as the free standing University of Medicine and Dentistry of New

Jersey, giving it the freedom to grow and be managed relatively free from the bureaucratic constraints of Trenton.

Anyone who could manage to survive the politically sensitive position of UMDNJ President with frequently changing party dominance at the state level and five different governors of vastly different temperaments must merit our admiration, grudging or not. The ability to move ahead in such an environment is not based on the rigid adherence to certain high and immutable ethical principles. Neither Bergen nor anyone else in his position could have survived nor could the institution he headed have done so without making compromises and negotiating deals. The boards of trustees that existed during this time served more as a cheering squad rather than an oversight team. It was generally believed that Bergen always had them safely in his pocket.

Although we now view with alarm and even disgust the shenanigans that have occurred at such high levels within UMDNJ, to be fair one most also acknowledge the great accomplishments of the institution despite its predilection for various kinds of chicanery. A part of this must be attributed to the leadership of Cadmus and even more to Bergen during the formative years of the institution.

From what began as two relatively small new schools of medicine and dentistry there was created the largest free standing health center in the country with eight schools located on five campuses throughout the state. Included are two medical schools, an osteopathic school and a dental school. The University owns and operates one hospital in Newark and utilizes four others for teaching purposes. In Newark alone, in addition to the University Hospital, the New Jersey Medical School and the Dental School, there is a School of Nursing, a Graduate School of Biological Sciences, a School for Health Related Professions, a School of Public Health, a Doctors' Office Center and the George F. Smith Library. Recently added to these is a Cancer Center, a new Ambulatory Care Facility, a new addition to the dental school and a large apartment complex for the use of over 450 students, house staff and some faculty. In 2006 UMDNJ student enrollment was 5764 and undoubtedly the production of health care professionals over the years has made medical care in the state more available and of higher quality than in the past. The budget for fiscal year 2008 was 1.5 billion dollars.

Although starting from a low point at the time of the move to Newark, research funding from national and other sources has grown consistently in recent years. For the fiscal year of 2005 UMDNJ placed 68th among all research institutions, medical schools and otherwise. For the same period in terms of NIH awards to the 126 U.S. medical schools the New Jersey Medical School placed 64th with almost 56 million dollars awarded and the Robert

Wood Johnson Medical School placed 66th with almost 55 million dollars in awards from this source alone. Well into 2010 UMDNJ and its component institutions continue to attract large amounts of Federal research dollars.

The record of the institution has been particularly laudable in regard to race relations within the city of Newark and opening up the doors of opportunity to minorities. A Board of Concerned Citizens was formed to deal early on with racial friction and community complaints before they could mature into riots. The Newark Agreements, reached in 1968 after the 1967 riots opened up formerly all-white unions to blacks and Hispanics. Multiple programs have been initiated to attract and help prepare minority students for careers in medicine. Today UMDNJ – and especially the New Jersey Medical School – are among the highest rated institutions nationally in the recruitment of such students.

However, perhaps the most important outcome of these deliberations was the decision to build a new hospital to replace the outdated Martland Hospital (formerly Newark City Hospital). This is what has enabled the provision of first rate health care for residents of the community. Newark City Hospital had often been referred to as "the butcher shop" by local residents. No such remarks could ever be justly directed at the current hospital and its clinics.

Getting back to the problems reported by the Star-Ledger, the most stinging accusation for this writer was that concerning the payment of 6 million dollars over 4 years to 18 cardiology practitioners in the surrounding area to send patients requiring heart surgery to the University Hospital. The recipients of this largesse received appointments as clinical assistant professors for which no services were demanded and they received annual payments of from $50,000 to $150,000. It certainly stirred personal resentment to learn that doctors half my age and with none of my credentials in some cases were earning more as pocket money than I did as a full professor at the time of my retirement in 1997. Worse than this, however, was the recognition that the faculty itself for the first time was being implicated in the UMDNJ scandals. Before this we could look upon it all as business as usual for those pencil pushers in the administration. Now it hit very close to home; the ethical rot had penetrated to the core of the institution, its faculty.

Although there is no excuse for such actions under any circumstances it might help those not directly involved to understand what went on and why by offering some perspective. As a cardiologist and long-time faculty member at the medical school in Newark, I will attempt to provide this. We begin with a rule of thumb: the more often you perform a procedure , whether it is the painting of a room, the driving of a car, the removal of a gall bladder, or the bypassing of a narrowed coronary artery, the more proficient you are likely to become. Having a heart surgery program is not only prestigious for a hospital but also a money maker. But if as many hospitals were allowed to have such programs as they desired the state would, no doubt, be flooded with underutilized facilities with sub par performance.

In order to prevent the uncontrolled proliferation of such programs, the state of New Jersey some years ago set up a board to decide which hospitals that had no program might qualify in the future because of perceived needs and which hospitals that already had heart surgery programs had not been performing adequately in terms of numbers of procedures as well as results. I served on this committee for several years.

Periodically, when we reviewed the records supplied by the various hospitals, we would come to University Hospital in Newark where, invariably, the numbers turned out to be lower than the standards set. Why was this so?

For many years one University Hospital administration after another acted as if it was because we did not have a surgeon with enough star power and they squandered hundreds of thousands of dollars on individuals who, they thought, would have cardiac patients breaking down our doors to secure their services. What the administrators did not realize is that it is not the quality of the surgeons that determines the numbers of patients they will get but the number of referring cardiologists. In one successful hospital after another where one sees a thriving cardiac surgical program one can also see that there might be as many as 35, 40, or even 50 cardiologists with busy private practices referring patients to their surgical colleagues. At the New Jersey Medical School/University Hospital we rarely had more than six or eight full-time cardiologists on staff and never more than 10 or 12. Furthermore, because of teaching, research and administrative responsibilities we could not manage a large patient practice even if we wanted to.

Another problem was the patient population our hospital cared for in Newark. There was plenty of coronary heart disease but most of the patients we saw were at an end-stage of their disease following multiple myocardial infarctions, complicated by hypertension, diabetes and other problems beyond the reach of existing surgical intervention. Sadly, many Newark residents with coronary disease were found to be succumbing to sudden unexpected cardiac deaths outside of the hospital before any care could be provided.

As for attracting patients from the suburbs, despite the passage of considerable time from 1967 during which Newark remained at peace, especially during the 1992 post-Rodney King uprisings, suburbanites are still afraid to come to Newark. The year of 1967 still hangs like the proverbial albatross around our collective neck.

Why then, with each go-around did the state committee fail to discontinue the program at the medical school? It was because cardiac surgery was recognized as an important component in the general surgical teaching program. The absence of a cardiac surgical program would also negatively impact the medical cardiology program, making it less attractive to potential candidates for such fellowships. Lack of cardiac surgery and a flawed cardiology program would weaken both surgery and the whole department of medicine, which everyone agrees is the backbone of any medical school. What would happen then? A true domino effect that, in the interests of medical education within the state, the committee wished to avoid. Lastly, elimination of a cardiac surgical program at University Hospital would effectively deprive local residents totally dependent upon it from access to such care on the occasions when it was needed. Prior to the bribery scandal University Hospital had excellent cardiologists and surgeons to respond to the needs of education, research and patient care. Neither the students, house staff, faculty nor patients there deserved to be victimized by some sort of numbers game imposed externally or thought up as an illegal ploy from within.

A final point on cardiac surgery: newer developments affecting cardiac surgery will make it even more difficult for the University Hospital cardiac surgery program as well as others to thrive. As cardiologists are performing more balloon angioplasties and stent implantations – about a million a year –instead of referring such patients to the surgeons, the number of coronary by-pass procedures, the bread and butter of the surgeons until now, have plummeted as much as 50 to 75 percent in once busy surgical practices. Newer graduates from cardiothoracic training programs are unable to find positions and openings for such resident training, once the most highly prized in the surgical arena, are going unfilled. What this means for the future of cardiac surgery in this country is another concern for worry but beyond the scope of this paper.

As a result of all the negative disclosures at UMDNJ heads have rolled. The long standing UMDNJ Vice President for Legal Affairs, Vivian Sanks King was forced to resign along with two compliance officers. Dr. Gallagher at the Osteopathic school and State Senator Bryant were found guilty of corruption charges. In July of 2009 Bryant was sentenced to four years in federal prison and forced to pay $113,167 in restitution to UMDNJ along with a fine of $25,000. In addition to this he was denied his full state pension of $84,000 annually. Gallagher received a prison sentence of one-and-a-half years along with $128,167 in financial penalties. The unscrupulous cardiologists who practiced play for pay are being pursued in the courts and three have already agreed to pay a combined $960,000, representing twice the amount that they had received from UMDNJ.

Five members of the Board of Trustees were soon replaced. Dr. Bergen's successor as president, a highly respected neurologist, Stuart D. Cook, managed to complete his term in 2004 before the current storm broke and was able to turn his full efforts once again to the neurosciences department at the New Jersey Medical School. Following him as President of UMDNJ, John Petillo was forced out following the virtual stockpiling of abuses and Bruce C. Vladeck, who then came in as acting president and who had hopes of succeeding him was convinced not to try.

In my own bailiwick, the Department of Medicine, the chairman, Dr. Jerrold Ellner was forced to resign both his chairmanship at the medical school and his position as chief of medicine in University Hospital. Although he must have shared in some responsibility for the cardiology fiasco, the possibility exists that he was made a scapegoat. It is unlikely that he was the instigator of the plan in the first place. An infectious disease specialist with special interests in AIDS and tuberculosis he is an international figure who had 29 million dollars in NIH grants coming along with him from his former position at Case-Western Reserve. It is not unreasonable to suppose that his mind as well as his body were frequently absent from the goings on in cardiology at University Hospital. An acting chairman has been in place since his departure and no permanent replacement is in sight as of mid 2010.

One encouraging act of retribution concerns the fate of a prominent whistle blower in this affair. Whereas so often such individuals wind up as victims rather than heroes, a faculty member who informed federal authorities of UMDNJ's double billing of Medicare and Medicaid, Steven Simring, received $800,000 out of a two million dollar settlement in a civil suit against UMDNJ. Although Simring, a former associate professor of psychiatry at the New Jersey Medical School, is no longer a faculty member, he continues on apparently unimpeded in his private practice.

Where do we stand now with the governance of UMDNJ? The former Board of Trustees was replaced by one little changed in character from its predecessor. Among the reconstituted board of 23 members there were four lawyers, down from seven. (Where were they all when they were needed?) There were three MDs, three dentists and an osteopath. The rest appeared to be business people, a number of them with connections to the pharmaceutical or medical instrument industries. There was no faculty representation on the previous board and this still remains the case.

It was not always thus. When I was president of the faculty I was invited to attend meetings of the Board of Trustees *ex officio* and allowed to make comments when I thought they were warranted. Following my term of office this invitation was withdrawn from future faculty representatives. After all, what do faculty know about running a medical school? What do doctors know about running a hospital? In this, our board is probably like most other university boards of trustees, filled with lawyers and businessmen who, we are told, know what it is to meet a payroll and are more competent than we to "keep an eye on the bottom line." But it seems the financial bottom line became blurred at UMDNJ and the ethical one crossed over too many times.

Our UMDNJ trustees are probably neither worse nor better than those calling the shots elsewhere. They are simply part of the subculture – or, more accurately in my view, a *supraculture* of privilege who become detached from the very people and institutions for which they are responsible. And it is in the arrogance of this isolation that they not only allow acts of dishonesty, but may encourage them and, at times, commit them. In a way the scandal at UMDNJ was only a curtain raiser to the much greater disaster in the financial markets that was to come in 2007 and 2008.

Getting back to UMDNJ, the selection of a new president, who began work in July of 2007, reflected the basic malaise of the whole system. One would have thought that, given the many recent missteps we have made, only the most squeaky clean of candidates would have made the cut. Although Dr. William F. Owen, Jr., who came to us from his position as chancellor of the Health Science Center of the University of Tennessee, is obviously intelligent, a first-rate clinician/researcher and probably a good administrator, he did not arrive with a completely unblemished reputation. According to the Star-Ledger, while at Tennessee he was prone to minor abuses of perks and prerogatives, fortunately not as great as those that have occurred among our higher echelon administrators in New Jersey. These have been explained away or brushed aside with statements to the effect that all this was just due to a misunderstanding and that amends were made. However, when all is said and done, one might ask if there exists *any* potential leader out there who is immune to the temptations at the top of overreaching their authority. We can only hope that the new president, chastened by his own personal peccadilloes in the past and well aware of the ethical minefield that he has now entered, will be able to lead his future board and the institution it represents into a new era of responsibility and accomplishment. His official swearing-in ceremony which finally took place in May 2009, nearly two years after his arrival, gives us hope that he is well on the way to doing just this.

Looking back on this whole mess one might ask what role we, as individuals, might have in perpetuating such scandals or, more important, preventing them. One recalls the dictum of that great Scottish historian, Thomas Carlyle: Make yourself an honest man and then you may be sure there is one less scoundrel in the world.

Perhaps if enough of us tried much harder to do so we might bring about some much needed change. But I wouldn't bet on it.

14

GREEK, LATIN, ENGLISH AND
ALL THAT:
THE LANGUAGES WE LIVE IN

I ONCE HAD A MEDICAL colleague who was a medievalist. By this I do not mean to imply that he was an expert on this historical period but rather that his mindset was firmly grounded in the Middle Ages. It was not that he held a personal grudge against the twentieth century; he just didn't think it was a very good idea.

I had no doubts about his being well versed in modern medicine, but at the end of the working day he would quickly disappear from the hospital scene and, I imagined, return to his local cloister for an evening meal on wooden or pewter plates. I then envisioned him humming Gregorian chants in the shower (if he had one) before snuffing out the candles and retiring to a bed of straw for the night. Considering his views on the true basis of meaningful civilization it was only natural that he was well-versed in both classic Greek and Latin and that he considered no one identifiable as an educated person who did not possess such qualifications.

Never having studied either Greek or Latin, I was always in awe of such true scholars who did. For years I lived in fear of one day being accosted by one of these classical dons who, spewing pure Plato out of one side of his mouth and Cicero out the other to my utter incomprehension, would effect my complete mortification.

Although I rejected the classic languages in favor of French as a New York City junior high school student in the 1940's it was not without a feeling of inadequacy as I recalled my father recounting his own high school experiences in the American backwater of West New York, New Jersey, where classroom conversations in Latin were routinely conducted. I was also in awe of my wife and her brothers who attended Swiss schools in Europe during their early years and were required to study Latin, which they actually enjoyed! To this day my better half extols the logic and comprehensiveness of Latin grammar. It appears that there is no human expression, no matter how noble or how vile, for which the Romans did not invent a declension.

Given the current dominance of English, it may be difficult to appreciate that not too long ago the study of Greek and Latin, now on the wane, were considered an integral part of a first rate education. For example, in Lytton Strachey's popular *Eminent Victorians,* first published in 1918, we find expressions in Greek appearing within the book without any translations provided.[1] Obviously the author assumed that any one intelligent enough to pick up his book would have no need for such assistance.

While the classics formed the bedrock of a proper education for many hundreds of years, it could be overdone. In the case of Anglo-American education there was an inordinate emphasis upon the classics in Victorian times in the English public schools ("private" in Americanese) where such knowledge was deemed paramount. That paradigm of pedagogy at Rugby, Dr. Thomas Arnold, who took over as headmaster in 1827, opined, "The study of language seems to me as if it was given for the very purpose of forming the human mind in youth; and the Greek and Latin languages seem the very instruments by which this is to be effected."[2]

While arguably valuable in educating the young, such intense study of the classics crowded out potentially important subjects that, to the modern mind, might reasonably be thought to have been useful. At Rugby the subject of history was limited to one hour a week; physical science was not taught at all. No doubt similar instruction regimens were in place at other public schools in Great Britain as well as elite private schools in the United States attempting to emulate them. One wonders about the aptness of that famous remark by the Duke of Wellington, "The battle of Waterloo was won on the playing fields of Eton." Perhaps that was because so little of real practical value was going on in the public school classrooms of the period.

This emphasis on the classics was carried into the higher reaches of British education as well, and had a particularly adverse effect on the study of medicine. Throughout the eighteenth century at Oxford and Cambridge study of the classics preempted an adequate medical curriculum and many of those aspiring to a career in medicine left England for Scotland or the continent to receive sufficient scientific training.[3] During the nineteenth and even the early twentieth century the study of scientific medicine in England was still hampered by, among other factors, the continued stranglehold of the classics upon university education.[4,5]

An example of this has been provided by Prof. W.F. Bynum, a distinguished medical historian, in describing the requirements for membership in the Royal College of Physicians in the mid nineteenth century when the oral examination was conducted in Latin and when "...the most ambitious candidates could have responded to the challenge of translating a Greek passage into Latin, a Latin passage into French, a French passage into German and a German passage into French."[6] Little wonder that succeeding generations of physicians attempted to escape such linguistic tyranny. During most of the Christian era the influence of Latin was more profound than that of Greek. It was, after all, the language of the Catholic Church. It was also a vital means of communication between scholars of the period, much in the way English, for all intents and purposes, became in the twentieth century. As useful as Latin may have been for international scientific communication – in Europe at least – early on there were pressures exerted in favor of the vernacular, especially beginning in the sixteenth century. These were preceded by the introduction of the printing press with Gutenberg's Bible in 1454, which certainly made the dissemination of information enormously more efficient in the years that followed. Galileo, who made his major discoveries in astronomy between 1610 and 1634, in order to make them more widely known published many of his findings in Italian as well as Latin – at least until the Inquisition got on his case.

As an occasional medical historian, I take particular interest in the role of linguistics as it applies to medical research and education. It is noteworthy that the great Swiss physician, Paracelsus (1493-1541) actually published in German and the equally great French military surgeon Ambroise Paré (1510-1590) also recorded his accomplishments in his native tongue. The real push for publication in the vernacular began at the beginning of the eighteenth century, by the end of which practically all medical papers were being published in the native language of the authors. With the blossoming of European medical research in the nineteenth and twentieth centuries the need for English speakers attempting to keep up with the literature became not a knowledge of Greek or Latin as much as French, German and Italian as the greater part of important research continued emanating from those countries at least until the beginning of the second World War.

In the United States much has been made of the requirement at the opening of the Johns Hopkins University School of Medicine that applicants planning to be part of the first class entering in 1893 have a reading knowledge of French and German and how this was considered a burden by many potential applicants thereafter. But at Harvard Medical School as far back as 1877 a reading knowledge of Latin, French or German was demanded of applicants and at Yale in 1900 exposure to Latin was still obligatory for those wishing to enter the medical school. Such requirements among these top institutions have disappeared along with those at any other medical school in the United States as well as the United Kingdom, as best as I have been able to determine. All that seems to remain of Latin are the names still appended to parts of human anatomy and some vestigial Latin abbreviations still employed by physicians in writing prescriptions .

Some medical educators have protested that this trend has gone too far, most notably Saul Jarcho (1906-2000) (see chapter 6), a natural linguist who was proficient in German, French, Italian, Latin, Hebrew and Arabic as well as English. In an editorial published in 1989 he decried the deterioration of linguistic skills among historical scholars. "In studying the history of medicine American nonphysician scholars share with physician scholars the disability that has been caused by American education, our great national failure. Unable to read Greek, Latin, Arabic and the languages of modern Europe, they are debarred from access to large parts of the clinical record."[7]

Although berating such individuals for lacking a knowledge of Arabic might seem a bit excessive for anyone but a gifted polyglot like Jarcho, his sentiments were and are shared, to some degree at least, by a number of others involved with the practice and teaching of medical history. In a more recent public comment on the reduction of language requirements by departments of history awarding Ph.D.s, the authors at the American Historical Association plaintively wrote, "We regret that the acquisition of a foreign language is now treated, especially in the American field, as a hurdle rather than a resource."[8]

Regarding the linguistic ability of modern physicians, Jarcho's case was not an isolated one. The heart surgeon, Michael E. DeBakey, while a medical student at Tulane during the 1930s, thanks to his cosmopolitan Lebanese background, could read the French and German medical literature of the time.[9] He got an important leg up in his academic career when the distinguished New Orleans surgeon Rudolph Matas learned of this student who was borrowing foreign language journals from his private library to translate articles for members of the faculty. Matas and then Alton Ochsner, who founded the famous clinic bearing his name, took DeBakey under their professional wings and sent him off for study at European centers of surgical research.

Paul Dudley White will be remembered by the general public as the cardiologist who cared for President Dwight D. Eisenhower when he suffered a coronary attack while in office. But he was much more than that. He was not only a leading practitioner of his specialty but a remarkable scholar. The bibliography of the first edition of his textbook (1931) contains over three thousand references.[10] Among these are 615 either in French or German and over 60 more in various other European languages. In a footnote to this massive compilation White confesses that there were actually 11 references that he had not read personally.

My own attempt to determine how much this familiarity with non-English sources of medical history has changed took the form of determining the changing linguistic sources of the references noted in articles published in the highly esteemed journal covering the field, the *Bulletin of the History of Medicine*. The study involved examining 100 full length articles from an earlier period (1939-1942) and comparing the languages used in their references with those represented in the references from 100 articles published in a more recent period (2000-2005). The results are indicated in Table 14.1. First off, it is obvious that the depth of documentation in more recent publications has increased markedly with the total number of references more than doubling. Equally striking is the fact that most of this increase has been in English language sources with an increase from 50 to 84 percent while the percent of Greek plus Latin references plummeted from 14 to 2 percent. There was also a marked decrease in the "other foreign languages" category (mostly French, German and Spanish) from 36 percent to 14 percent. The increasing preoccupation with Anglo-American subject matter for research is reflected in an increase of the number of papers devoted to this from 28 to 60 percent. Papers with only English references increased from 18 to 28 percent. The same scrutiny of papers published in the British-based journal *Medical History* provided similar although less striking results.

Table 14.1. Articles from *The Bulletin of the History of Medicine*

	Anglo-American Subjects	Total Refs.	English Only	Distribution Total Refs. (%) English Greek/ Latin Others
1939-1942 (n=100)	28	3477	18	1739 487 1251 (50) (14) (36)
2000-2005 (n=100)	60	7919	28	6652 158 1109 (84) (2) (14)

English only = number of articles with references only from English language sources; Others = predominantly French, German, Spanish and Italian sources.

Those more sanguine about such trends than critics like Jarcho might imply that formal language study for those planning to do medical history research is not really necessary: the researcher can pick up the language involved with a particular investigation when and if necessary.

Of course someone working on the history of the medical schools in Padua or Bologna would certainly not embark on such a project without learning Italian and probably Latin. For someone investigating the growth of laboratory medicine in central Europe during the nineteenth century a knowledge of German would be absolutely essential and so on. But such a utilitarian approach to language misses the point. Educators all encourage the study of geometry and algebra in our schools not because our children are headed for careers in architecture or engineering, but because the study of mathematics hones the minds of these students so that they may become more analytical in their thinking over a wide range of life's problems and experiences. Similarly, the study of languages is not just a career tool; it strengthens the underpinnings of our intellect so that we can better understand the world around us, especially the more distant parts and the cultures they contain.

The rapid emergence of English as the *lingua franca* of the modern world in the twenty-first century threatens to obliterate such otherwise worthy cultural goals. It has been estimated that among the 6.5 billion inhabitants on earth 1.6 billion (roughly 25 percent) use English as their primary, secondary or tertiary language.[11]

This goes far beyond those parts of the world described as Anglo-American. When I visited China for the first time over 20 years ago and was besieged by friendly youths asking to practice their English with me, I was told that there were more Chinese studying English than there were citizens of the United States. Since then the numbers have undoubtedly increased. When I once asked an Indian in Mumbai (Bombay) about her assessment of the British rule in her country she replied, "They took a lot but they gave a lot." Not the least part of that legacy was the language that has been the glue holding together otherwise diverse societies making up the most populous democracy in the world. A recent consensus held that about a third of the Indian population, about 350 million, were capable of carrying on a conversation in English, on a par with the current United States population.[12] (Incidentally, Nehru, who often talked in his sleep, reportedly did so in English.)

Much to the chagrin of the French, who held a virtual monopoly on the language of international diplomacy for many years, English is now becoming dominant in such affairs as well as displacing French in the European Union.[13] We learned some years ago from Robert MacNeil's television series, "The Story of English," that the trend was already sky borne: all over the world, whenever an international flight approaches an airport for a landing the pilots and air traffic controllers communicate in English.

The current trend toward English as the new *lingua franca* of the world should carry with it a caution. It can lead to a certain smugness among the English speaking peoples that might easily degenerate into a kind of linguistic xenophobia. The ubiquity of English may be useful but that does not mean that it should be exclusive. There should be no barriers toward any foreign "contamination" of a particular country's "sacred tongue." The French academics' resistance to *Franglais* is a prime example of such foolish and ultimately futile antics. At home in the United States we have the movement to make English the official language under law. Although such efforts may relieve our legislators of having to concentrate on such other distractions as Iraq, Afghanistan, the ballooning national debt, economic recession, health care and global warming, it is not clear to what extent, if any, this might affect the adoption of English by the "invading hoards" of new immigrants. As with former newcomers, they will learn some basic English, not out of patriotic ardor but rather because they realize that this is the key to economic opportunity and better futures for themselves and their families. Their children will, no doubt, be perfectly at home with English and some of their grandchildren will probably be pursuing Ph.D.s in it at select universities.

How has English dominance impacted on language study in higher education? A recent article based on data from the National Center for Education Statistics noted that in the United States, "There are more bachelor degrees awarded every year in Parks, Recreation, Leisure and Fitness Studies than in all foreign languages and literatures combined."[14] This certainly bodes ill for the future literacy of our college graduates. Hope, however, looms on the horizon.

It is in the pre-college years, primarily, that a recent revival of interest in foreign languages is being manifested. Throughout the land those whose parents, when they attended public schools, were severely reprimanded for using the language of their own forbears such as French Canadians in Maine, are now encouraging their own children to incorporate such a valued linguistic heritage into their own daily lives.[15] Notable efforts are being made for Yiddish and the study of Gaelic is blooming in Irish-speaking schools and universities.[16] Nursery schools featuring the teaching of Chinese are becoming big business not only for ethnic Chinese-Americans but also for other Westerners with entrepreneurial aims if not cultural ones, who want their kids exposed to Mandarin as China emerges as an economic powerhouse in the twenty-first century.

In the meantime, choice expressions in French, German, Italian, Yiddish and other languages will continue to enrich our written and spoken dialogue. This has been amply demonstrated in the growing sophistication and internationalization of the winning words of the present compared with those of the past in the Scripps National Spelling Bee. Back in the twenties readily recognized words like gladiolus, cerise, luxuriance and albumen took the prize. Over the last ten years the foreign derivations are more obscure but strikingly connected with their sources by pronunciation as well as origin: Italian (pococurante, appoggiatura); Greek (autochthonous); Latin (succedaneum); French (demarche, guerdon); and German (Ursprache). In 2010 the two final correctly spelled words that led to the prize were *juvia* (a Brazil nut, Spanish and Portuguese in derivation) and *stromuhr* (a tool for measuring blood flow, Germanic in origin).

Where does this leave the teaching of Greek and Latin, the subject that gave rise to this essay in the first place?

In the United Kingdom it appears that the Arnold tradition, in more realistic dosages, is being upheld. At both Rugby and Eton Latin is currently a required course while the study of Greek is optional. Such steadfastness is also reflected in American counterparts of such institutions. At Groton two years of Latin or Greek are required in addition to a modern language, with many students choosing to extend their classical studies beyond the minimum. At Choate-Rosemary Hall (the school is now co-educational) Latin and Greek are both offered on a voluntary basis and appear to be popular with the student body.

It is in the American public school arena that perhaps even more noteworthy developments are taking place. At Boston Latin, the oldest public school in the United States (founded 1635) three to four years of Latin are still compulsory and Greek is offered as an elective. In New York City, where the schools always seem to be in a swirl of reorganization lately, a Brooklyn Latin School opened its doors in September 2006 in emulation of its Boston antecedent. Elsewhere in the city among its over 300 high schools Latin is offered in about a fifth of them and Greek taught in eight.

On the national scene the American Council on the Teaching of Foreign Languages keeps a tab on such developments over time and published their last report in 2002.[17] Over the years although the study of Greek indeed seems to have gone into decline, Latin has had its ups and downs. In 1900, although only 500,000 public students studied foreign languages, 51 percent were enrolled in Latin classes. By 1948 this had fallen to 8 percent and in 2000 had bottomed out at 1.3 percent. In 2010 the situation remains unchanged. On the brighter side, in 2006 143,000 students elected to take the National Latin Examination. And while Spanish and French continue to be the most popular languages studied, it appears now that Latin is edging out German for the third most popular language in the hearts and minds of our high school students.

What could all this mean? Could some of these findings actually signal a revival of the classical tradition as well as a renewed appreciation of more modern foreign languages? And is English capable of accommodating such a resurgence?

RES IPSA LOQUITUR.

ACKNOWLEDGMENTS: Many individuals with various institutional affiliations were kind enough to assist the author with pertinent information. Among them were: Martha G. Abbott (American Council on the Teaching of Foreign Languages); Tad R. Bennicoff (Princeton University); Peter Cohee (Boston Latin School); Rick Connors (Groton School); Judy Donald (Choate-Rosemary Hall); Jack Eckert (Harvard University); Gerard Evans (Eton College); Eric V.D. Luft (SUNY Upstate, Syracuse); Andrew Maynard (Eton College); Jeremy Norman (Norman Publishing); Michael J. North (National Library of Medicine); Henry Price (Rugby School); Ron Woo (New York City Board of Education); and Mary Yearl (Yale University).

REFERENCES

1. Strachey L. *Eminent Victorians. 4*[th] *Impression.* New York:Capricorn Books, 1963.

2. Ibid pp 208-209.

3. Bonner TN. *Becoming a Physician. Medical Education in Great Britain, France, Germany and the United States 1750-1945.* Oxford: Oxford Univ. Press, 2005. p 40.

4. Ibid. p. 183.

5. Henderson J. *A Life of Ernest Starling.* Oxford: Oxford Univ. Press, 2005.

6. Bynum WF. Practicing on principles. Medical textbooks in 19th century Britain. The Nineteenth John H. McGovern Lecture. Delivered before the American Osler Society, April 29, 2004, Houston, Texas.

7. Jarcho S. Some observations and opinions on the present state of American historiography. *J Hist Med & Allied Sci* 1989 44:288-290.

8. Bender T, Katz PM Palmer C and the Committee on Graduate Education of the American Historical Association. *The Education of Historians for the Twenty-first Century.* Urbana:Univ. of Illinois Press , 2004, p. 57.

9. DeBakey ME. In Weisse AB. *Heart to Heart. The Twentieth Century Battle Against Cardiac Disease. An Oral History.* New Brunswick: Rutgers Univ. Press, 2002. pp 181-182.

10. White PD. *Heart Disease.* New York: MacMillan, 1931.

11. Crystal D. *The Cambridge Encyclopedia of the English Language. 2*[nd] *Edition.* Cambridge:Cambridge Univ. Press 2003. pp 106-108.

12. Crystal D. Personal communication 2007.

13. Tagliabue J. Soon Europe will speak in 23 tongues. New York Times, Dec. 6, 2006, p.A8.

14. Menand L. The New Yorker Magazine. May 21, 2007, pp 27-28.

15. Belluck P. Long scorned in Maine, French has a Renaissance. New York Times, June 4, 2006, National Report, p. 26.

16. Lavery B. Irish tongues are wagging in U.S. classrooms. New York Times, June 14, 2006. Metro Section B9.

17. Draper JB, Hicks JH. Foreign language enrollments in public secondary schools, Fall 2000. American Council on the Teaching of Foreign Languages, 2002.

15

A Fond Farewell to the Foxglove ?
The Decline in the Use of Digitalis

IT WAS NOT UNTIL the beginning of the twentieth century that physicians could express some well-founded confidence in the effectiveness of some of our therapeutic agents. This was best expressed by Lawrence J. Henderson (1878-1942) who is credited with the statement that "Somewhere between 1910 and 1912 in this country a random patient with a random disease consulting a doctor chosen at random had, for the first time in the history of mankind, a better than fifty-fifty chance of profiting from the encounter."[1] The sad state of medical therapy before this had been commented on earlier by Oliver Wendell Holmes (1809-1894) in one of his essays on medical science: "I firmly believe that if the whole materia medica *as now used* could be sunk to the bottom of the sea, it would be all the better for mankind – and all the worse for the fishes."[2]

The popularity of homeopathy during the nineteenth century was probably related to the fact that the miniscule doses of medicines prescribed by the adherent physicians protected their patients from the all too often occurring toxic effects of many of the medicines popular during this period. The great William Osler (1849-1919) was well aware of the uselessness of many of the medicines recommended during his life time as well as their frequent toxicity. He had no qualms about being branded as a "therapeutic nihilist" because of his reluctance to dispense many of the medicines in vogue during his time.[3] One of the rare exceptions to his exclusionary approach to medications was digitalis. Osler's most distinguished protégé, George Dock, was also a skeptic. He would tell his students that he was guided by the expression that a young physician has 20 remedies for every disease while an older one has 20 remedies for all diseases.[4] However, in his list of 20 for 1900 he included digitalis, which has survived in popularity for many years while the use of such nostrums such as arsenic, strychnine, calomel and balsam, included in his lists, has faded.

The enthusiasm for digitalis has been on the wane, which comes as something of a surprise for older physicians who grew up professionally when digitalis was looked upon as a strong ally when it came to treating congestive heart failure as well as controlling ventricular rate in atrial fibrillation. Fifty years ago our therapeutic arsenal was rather limited when it came to other drugs of use in these conditions. Besides digitalis there was quinidine, of course, and then the invaluable mercurial diuretics which had been introduced in the 1920s and little else.

So dependent were physicians upon the use of digitalis in heart disease that its administration became something of an institution in itself, perhaps even an art form for those who used to wield it in pursuit of therapeutic success. A half century ago rapid digitalization was frequently achieved with lanatoside-C (Cedilanid) administered intravenously. Several oral forms were in general use. Physician preference depended upon differences in absorption, persistence of effect and propensity for inducing toxicity. Digitoxin, digoxin and digitalis leaf were the major contenders and supporters of each could resemble religious zealots in their differing advocacies. Digitoxin attracted adherents because it was fully absorbed from the gut perhaps making loading dosages more predictable. Because of its longer lasting effect it was argued that patients would not lose digitalization if they forgot to take their daily dose. On the other hand, cases of digitalis toxicity induced by digitoxin would be more prolonged than with digoxin. Digoxin is only 50 to 80% absorbed and this variability put off some practitioners. It was shorter lasting than digitoxin: although patients might become under digitalized by failing to take their daily dose they would benefit by a more rapid recovery should toxicity occur. A cruder preparation, digitalis leaf, was favored by some because they thought that the effects of over dosage on the stomach might precede the centrally induced vomiting and potentially lethal effects of over dosage on cardiac rhythm.

Whatever preparation a physician favored he was admonished to be expert in its utilization and the importance of digitalis was rarely questioned. If you knew how to use digitalis, in whatever form you preferred, you knew just about all you could about treating heart failure and atrial fibrillation.

Over the years digoxin won out among the available oral preparations and, when digitalis is used today it is this formulation that cardiologists and others employ. But even this form of the drug seems to be losing out to other medications with which we have been blessed in treating both heart failure and atrial fibrillation. Angiotensin converting enzyme (ACE) inhibitors, angiotensin receptor blockers, beta blockers, aldosterone antagonists and a variety of new potent diuretics have eliminated mercurials from the formulary and seriously question the use of digitalis as well.

A detailed review of the extensive literature concerning the use of digitalis in current medical practice is beyond the scope of this paper. However, a few observations may be in order.

In atrial fibrillation, where ventricular rate control is a major aim of therapy use of digitalis in recent years has been discounted because of the general impression that, although rate can be well controlled at rest, with exercise this may not be the case.[5] Nonetheless, in the AFFIRM Study (The Atrial Fibrillation Follow-up Investigation of Rhythm Management) in which efficacy of rate control at rest and exercise with three different drugs, singly or in combination, was evaluated, digoxin alone had a 58 % success rate compared with beta blockers (59 %) and calcium channel blockers (38 %).[6] The highest rates of success (70-78 %) were achieved by digoxin in combination with one or two of the other drug classes.

The reputation of digitalis in the treatment of congestive heart failure (CHF) has also suffered in recent years. In the 2005 guidelines of the American Heart Association and the American College of Cardiology for the treatment of CHF digitalis is barely mentioned.[7] Two years later a published round table discussion of the treatment of acute heart failure none of the experts even mentioned digitalis.[8] For many cardiologists the report of the Digitalis Investigation Group that appeared in 1997 was a final confirmation of digitalis's lack of effectiveness.[9] In this large study of over 6000 patients CHF characterized by low ejection fractions ("systolic failure") digitalis added to other medications had no effect on mortality; and this seemed to settle the matter in many minds. Other important findings, such as digitalis reducing need for hospitalization or reducing the progression of heart failure, were generally overlooked. Also noteworthy are the findings of other studies released about the time of the Digitalis Investigation Group report showing the benefits of digitalis in CHF even with patients in sinus rhythm, a group traditionally thought poorly responsive to such treatment.[10-12]

Given such findings as well as new knowledge about the metabolism of digoxin, the ability to measure serum levels and the ability to treat digitalis intoxication now with specific antibodies to digoxin all make a case against the premature rejection of its role in the treatment of CHF.

The demonstrable utility of digitalis notwithstanding, there seems to have been an undeniable decline in its clinical use. By 2007-08 it was no longer one of the ten most popular drugs prescribed by cardiologists.[13] (Multiple attempts by the author to obtain further quantitative information on production and sales of digitalis preparations from pharmaceutical manufacturers were unsuccessful.)

Such ruminations about the current status of digitalis lead back to a reconsideration of the source of its reputation as one of the great botanical gifts to mankind for over two hundred years.[14] William Withering's own words about his discovery still ring familiar to many of today's physicians: "In the year 1775 my opinion was asked concerning a family receipt for the cure of the dropsy. I was told that it had long been kept a secret by an old woman in Shropshire who had sometimes made cures after regular practitioners had failed…This medicine was composed of twenty or more different herbs; but it was not difficult for one *conversant in these subjects* [italics added] to perceive that the active herb could be no other than the Foxglove."

How many modern physicians, learning of some miracle cure of an obscure person in the hinterlands with a concoction of 20 different herbs, would have the slightest idea of how to go about determining what the active ingredient might be? The fact is that many of the 18th century medicines available to physicians of the period were derived from native plants and it was the practitioners' duty to be aware of them. Withering, in particular, was well grounded in botany. He had long been an enthusiast about the subject and at the time of his first encounter with the the foxglove as a therapeutic agent he had already published a massive highly acclaimed study on the plant life of Great Britain.[15]

Before Withering's use of foxglove in dropsy it had been used as a remedy for various other disorders. Among them foxglove was used as a purgative to empty the bowels although its action as an emetic was much more pronounced and a more constant sign of toxicity when this occurred. Withering's great insight was contained in a sentence omitted from the previous quote: "I was informed also that the effects produced were violent vomiting and purging; for the *diuretic effects* [italics added] seemed to have been overlooked."

By focusing on the amount of urine produced by treatment with digitalis rather than on the expulsion of fluids either through vomiting or diarrhea, Withering was able to establish the usefulness of the active principle he extracted from the foxglove. For those who are of the impression that this was an epiphany occurring over a short span of time, reference to his original report will show that it consisted of 207 pages of carefully accumulated documentation obtained over a ten year period (1775-1785).

As one reads through this remarkable document Withering's pharmaceutical skills were as impressive his medical ones. Perhaps, being the son of a successful apothecary exposed Withering to some of this methodology. He determined that it was the leaves of the plant rather than the roots, stems, flowers or seeds that contained the active principle. He noted a seasonal variation in the strength of the drug in the powder he prepared from the leaves. He prepared different forms of the drug for administration to his patients, as a liquid ("infusion") or making up pills by incorporating the powder in soap or gum ammoniac.

At first he prescribed the drug to the point of vomiting but later realized that an adequate diuresis could be achieved before this toxic manifestation occurred. He determined which types of cases were more likely to respond : e.g. those with hydrothorax (pleural effusions) which were often likely due to congestive heart failure and those that would not : those with ovarian cysts, consumption or hydrocephalus.

Some have suggested that Withering was ignorant of the mechanism of foxglove's action. On the contrary, while he never once mentions the kidneys, in his section entitled "Inferences" toward the end of his monograph he states "That it has a power over the motion of the heart, to a degree yet unobserved in any other medicine, and that this power may be converted to salutary ends." Finally, in describing the toxic effects of the drug other than vomiting he notes the disturbances of vision (green or yellow) as well as what was probably advanced heart block by detecting a pulse rate of 40 in a patient (#106) who had been overdosed. All these findings as a result of over dosage have been confirmed time and time again throughout the history of the drug.

How well did Withering's foxglove perform? He describes 163 cases in widely varying detail; some case reports occupy several pages, while 25 consist of 5 lines or less. I attempted to determine success according to diagnosis, seeking to separate out those who, to this cardiologist, were almost undoubtedly suffering from CHF from the rest with other etiologies of their dropsy (e.g. liver disease, kidney disease, ovarian cysts and possibly intra-abdominal cancers). The identification of those most likely to have heart disease depended mainly on history, symptomatology and the presence of pleural effusions ("hydrothorax"). Since this work was all done pre-Laennec there were no auscultatory findings to provide such leads as to causation. Pulse rate was noted infrequently and blood pressure, of course, was not measured at all.

Eleven cases were eliminated from this analysis by the author for lack of sufficient information to suggest either cardiac or other causes of dropsy. The results among the remaining 152 patients were favorable in 64 % (98/152). When those identified as most likely to have been in heart failure were separated out (Table 15.1) the success rate rose to 89%. Considerable success among the others (55 %) no doubt indicates a number of cardiac cases among them, not meeting the rather strict criteria adopted for this analysis.

Table 15.1. Withering's success in treating dropsy: 152 cases.

Patients	Success (%)	Failure	Total
Definite Cardiac	39(89)	5	44
Others	59(55)	49	108

Were such data presented in a paper submitted to any modern journal they would no doubt be immediately rejected. What did Withering know about a randomized, prospective double blind study to determine therapeutic efficacy? Fortunately for millions of patients over the last 200 years this was no impediment to his wonderful contribution.

REFERENCES

1. Blumgart HL. Caring for the patient. *New Engl J Med* 1964;270:449-456.

2. Holmes OW. *Currents and countercurrents in medical science In Medical Essays 1842-1882.* Boston:Houghton Mifflin, 1891, p. 203.

3. Osler W. An address on the treatment of disease. *Brit Med J* 1909;2:185-189.

4. Davenport HW. *Doctor Dock. Teaching and learning medicine at the turn of the century.* New Brunswick:Rutgers University Press, 1987, p.62.

5. Kay GN, Vance JP. Atrial fibrillation, atrial flutter and atrial tachycardia In *Hurst's the Heart 11ᵗʰ Edition.* Ed. Fuster V, Alexander RW, O'Rourke RA.. New York:McGraw Hill, 2004, 836-837.

6. Olshansky B, Rosenfield LE, Warner AL, Soloman AJ, O'Neill G, Sharma A, et al. The atrial fibrillation Follow-up investigation of rhythm management (AFFIRM) study. *J Am Coll Cardiol* 2004;43:1201-1208.

7. Hunt SA, Abraham WT, Chin MH, Feldman AM, Francis GH, Ganiats TG, et al. ACC/AHA 2005 guideline for the diagnosis and management of chronic heart failure in the adult. *Circulation* 2005;112:1825-1852.

8. Friedewald VE, Gheorghiade M, Yancy CW, Young JB, Roberts WC. The editor's roundtable: Acute decompensated heart failure. *Am J Cardiol* 2007;99:1560-1567.

9. Garg R, Gorlin R, Smith T, Yusuf S, The Digitalis Investigation Group. The effect of digoxin on mortality and morbidity in patients with heart failure. *New Engl J Med* 1997;336:525-533.

10. Packer M, Gheorghiade M, Young JB, Costantini PJ, Adams KF, Cody RJ, et al.. Withdrawal of digoxin from patients with chronic heart failure treated with angiotensin-converting enzyme inhibitors. *New Engl J Med* 1993;329:1-7.

11. Uretsky BF, Young JB, Shahidi FE, Yellen LG, Harrison MC, Jolly MK. Randomized study assessing the effect of digoxin withdrawal in patients with mild to moderate chronic congestive

heart failure: Results of PROVED trial. *J Am Coll Cardiol* 1993;22:955-962.

12. vanVeldhuisen DJ, deGraeff DA, Remme WJ, Lie KI. Value of digoxin in heart failure and sinus rhythm: New features for an old drug? *J Am Coll Cardiol* 1996;28:813-819.

13. Vital Signs. Top 10 drugs prescribed by cardiologists. *Cardiol News* 2008;6:1.

14. Recommended is Aronson's reproduction of the original report with marginal notations to guide the modern reader non-conversant with 18th century terms and concepts: Aronson JK. *An Account of the Foxglove and Its Medical Uses.* London:Oxford University Press, 1985.

15. Withering W. *A Botanical Arrangement of all the Vegetables Naturally Growing in Great Britain. 2 vols.* London:M Sivinney, 1776. 838 pp.

16

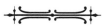

I Was a Mole in an IRB

If you haven't learned the difference between right and wrong by the age of 12 then you never will. (Anonymous)

THE MESSAGE BEHIND THIS seemingly homespun bit of folk wisdom is deceptive. It subtly implies that by the time of puberty we should all have obtained such knowledge. At the same time it tells us that for those who have failed in this respect no amount of remedial efforts to compensate for this will succeed. Evidence that right mindedness may not come with puberty abounds. We have only to recall that it was one of the most scientific and culturally advanced countries of Europe that gave us the Holocaust. The response to the medical atrocities it encompassed was the adoption of guidelines such as the Nuremburg Code (1945) and the Helsinki Declaration (1964) to insure the proper respect for and protection of patients participating in clinical research.

In the years following World War II with the rapid expansion of clinical research in this country different ethical challenges arose as it became apparent that such abuses of human research as lack of informed consent and insufficient protection of medical subjects were occurring. Examples of these were highlighted by the anesthesiologist Henry K. Beecher in a landmark article published in 1966.[1] An historical perspective of these problems was provided by David J. Rothman in his book *Strangers at the Bedside*.[2] In it he called the years 1966-1976 "the critical period of change" in clinical research, and outlined the rise of ethical standards to address the kinds of problems Beecher had earlier reported.

Although the Helsinki Code has been updated as recently as 2000 newer instruments of oversight have continued to emerge. For clinical investigators none of these have had as direct an impact upon the conduct of medical research in this country as the creation of the Institutional Review Board (IRB). Legally established by the National Research Act of 1974 and becoming operative in the 1980s with subsequent revisions, the system of IRBs has become the overseer of all who would attempt to conduct research involving humans in the United States.

Given the evidence of misdeeds in the past and the need to prevent them in the future it is difficult to oppose such monitoring. But how pertinent and how effective is it in practice? What follows is an account of one individual's experience with his local IRB and an extended attempt to understand its workings.

Having graduated medical school in 1958 and beginning both animal and human research in the 1960s I was able to perform a large body of my biological research outside the shadow of anything like an IRB. I believe my animal research was performed in full accordance with the guidelines of the American Physiological Society. The guidelines for my research with humans involved my own sense of ethics and decency. My first brush with the IRB at our institution came in the mid 1980s in connection with a grant proposal I had made to the National Institutes of Health (NIH) involving subjects with a particular kind of heart disease. I submitted a copy of the proposal to our recently established IRB. No fault was found with the rights or safety of the participating patients. However, what I did receive were objections to the research design; this from an IRB without any qualifications for making any such judgments. Naturally I was outraged. If my proposal had such defects the expert panel of reviewers at the NIH was perfectly capable of detecting them. As it turned out the issue became moot: like so many applications at the time my project was approved but not funded. Nevertheless my resentment of this overstepping of their authority by the IRB continued to fester.

My next encounter involved a book I was preparing, an oral history of twentieth century cardiology and cardiac surgery. A previous work covering a wider swath of twentieth century medicine had been published in 1984 with no repercussions.[3] The interviews conducted with leading medical figures who contributed were all published only after their full scrutiny and approval. All were pleased with the result which, incidentally, won an award as one of the outstanding books of this type for that year. My new work, begun almost twenty years later included some material from its predecessor as well as more recent interviews conducted throughout the country. To assist with travel expenses I applied for a small grant from the National Library of Medicine which was offering such support at the time to historical scholars. I sent a copy of the project proposal to our IRB, which insisted that I obtain informed consents from the contributors. My sense of outrage was reignited. First, such a requirement was obviously demeaning to the contributors suggesting that these seasoned outstanding scientists were incapable of recognizing if they were being drawn into some shady scam or not. Second, there was the oblique suggestion that I could be the potential perpetrator of such a nefarious scheme. Finally, by the time the series was completed in manuscript form some of the contributors had already died having previously given their personal approval to me. Would I now have to gain consent from their surviving families? What kind of a legal tangle might this possibly involve? I withdrew my application to the National Library of Medicine and published the book as an independent scholar rather than under the aegis of my medical school.[4] The book was heartily approved by all the contributors and their families.

At the time of my retirement from full-time academic status in 1997 one of my planned future projects was an assessment of the IRB system and its potential for inhibiting medical research and discouraging medical investigators. I finally got around to volunteering for my department early in 2007. I determined that the best way to accomplish this would be to insinuate myself within the ranks of the regulators and lie low for a time gathering the evidence. Then I would dramatically reveal my true crusading identity by unleashing an expose of what our IRB really was: the embodiment of a despotic bureaucracy run amok, throttling both scientific enterprise and innovation. It didn't quite turn out that way.

The first steps involved in the process turned out as onerous as I had anticipated. HIPAA (Health Insurance Portability and Accountability Act) credentialing was required. I was referred to a website where I took a brief course of instruction followed by a rather straightforward examination.

To prepare me for my duties as an IRB member I was supplied with two books. The first, at over 300 pages, was a manual covering all the issues coming under the purview of committees at investigative sites.[5] The other, somewhat more condensed and covering some similar ground was the IRB handbook.[6] After studying these I was directed to an Internet site for further instruction by the Protection of Human Research Participants (PHRP) Training Course. I was told this would take two to three hours; it took six. The course was followed by an examination consisting of multiple choice questions requiring an 80% passing rate. A recurring problem for me with the examination questions was deciding which of the answers to choose: the one I suspected they wanted or another that I thought would really be closer to the truth. I managed to get by with one correct answer over the minimum required, and was granted a Human Subject Protection certificate (HSP).

No sooner did I complete jumping through this hoop than I learned that a totally new course and examination would be required by December of 2007. This was CITI (the Collaborative IRB Training Initiative) a much more rigorous and in depth obstacle course than its predecessor. Preparatory study varies depending upon the role of the applicant. For an investigator in a particular field perhaps only 12 to 15 modules need to be successfully completed. For a member of an IRB board such as myself who might see a variety of different types of applications 31 modules needed to be completed with a matching set of questions that needed to be answered correctly following them. I decided to get this over with as soon as possible and started devoting the morning hours of each day to accomplish this. It took two weeks (ten mornings) before the task was over. Every three years, following a refresher course successful completion of another examination is required to maintain certification.

At least now I could take my place around the deliberative table. UMDNJ (the University of Medicine and Dentistry of New Jersey) is the largest free standing health care institution of its kind in the United States. Eight colleges of various types and five hospitals throughout the state operate under its banner. To handle the IRB load for UMDNJ throughout the state of New Jersey there are separate IRB centers in Newark, New Brunswick and Stratford. In Newark alone the work is divided among four separate groups. I was assigned to the Red Team. I was amazed to learn that the Newark IRB has oversight over 1200 grants each year, about a quarter of them being new applications. Regulations require that there be at least five members on a board representing both professional and community groups. I was pleased to see that there were about a dozen active members on the Red Team fairly equally divided between these two constituencies. Our professionals (e.g. MDs, PhDs, nurses etc.) were certainly adequately represented and, I soon observed, dominated most of the discussions.

The intensity with which each human research proposal is scrutinized depends upon its character. Certain types of research can be exempted from board approval or just undergo expedited review by an experienced IRB member if they involve minimal risk and, in most cases, no patient identifying features. It is the latter, I believe, that disqualifies most clinical investigators from attempting this route since many of us at one point or another anticipate the need to evaluate results in certain patients who have participated in a study. *Any* identifying feature – name, chart number, study number, social security number etc. – cannot be employed if exempt or expedited review is requested. As a result I believe the bulk of submissions involve full board approval and since annual reviews are usually required of studies in progress the work load is substantial. Incidentally, while an expedited review may take 10 to 14 days ordinarily, a full board review may take up to a month and a half or even longer. I remain uncertain about how this is all handled efficiently. I was encouraged to learn, however, that in the experience of one seasoned IRB official with over a decade long experience only one study had actually not been approved even after the IRB tried to work with the investigators. (Naturally, some research applications approved in terms of patient safety and confidentiality are not carried out due to ultimate failure to obtain funds from the granting agency involved.) Gradually I became convinced that the function of our IRB was ultimately to get the investigators over the hurdles and enable them to perform their work rather than stop them dead in their tracks.

For the first couple of months I acted mainly as an observer, more or less rubber stamping the recommendations of the more experienced members of the board. However, after all my studying and test passing - not to mention over three decades of conducting human research in a university setting – I was eager to assume a more active role as a primary reviewer. I was told that in the past new members, after observing a few sessions, were given test proposals and then critiqued to assure competence. This option was never made available to me. The prevailing view during my initiation seemed to be that a new board member just by sitting there for a year or so and observing the others could learn, supposedly by a process of osmosis, how to function more fully in the capacity of grant reviewer. I, for one, did not intend to sit there passively after all my preparation. I finally demanded to be given proposals to evaluate and after six months they began to come my way.

How well does an IRB function, at least the one I joined? Prior to each monthly meeting new or continuing applications for full board review are assigned to pairs of reviewers for in depth analysis and comment contained in written assessments. Copies of the applications, usually 6 to 12 at a sitting are distributed to other members of the board prior to the scheduled meeting. On the Red Team we had two internists/cardiologists, an anesthesiologist, a pathologist, a neurosurgeon, an ophthalmologist, a psychologist and a highly credentialed midwife. Thus technical details can usually be clarified for the benefit of the lay people on the board. When necessary, primary reviewers may contact the applicant directly for clarification or additional information prior to submitting his or her report but this is rarely necessary. I found the reviewers to be fair, hard working and dedicated. Despite their best efforts though, they as well as the applicants were hampered by the complicated and often confusing composition of the IRB forms. As a result of this almost invariably clerical errors were often detected. Fortunately these were usually of a minor nature and almost all applications could be approved pending minor revisions. Repeated attempts to clarify and refine the paperwork have been attempted but with only partial success. Despite this obstacle, during three years of service on the board, I witnessed no outright rejections.

One of the sore points mentioned above – and one that affected me directly – is the stated responsibility for IRBs to review the scientific content of proposals in addition to patient protection issues. I maintain that this is still inappropriate and that other reviewing bodies are more capable of performing this function. However, what happens when there are no expert extramural reviewing bodies to assess the scientific merit of a proposal? Recently we had a proposal, funded by a hospital department, to study some psychiatric aspects concerning the patients that came under their care. There were no co-investigators or consultants with any psychology or psychiatric credentials on board despite the possible risk of psychiatric side effects and the need for proper selection of psychiatric testing techniques. Even with such glaring deficiencies the proposal was not rejected but tabled pending further consultations with the department involved. Thus it seems that in some cases some intervention of an IRB regarding study plans might be fully justified

Other problems persist. Each hospital involved with clinical research has its own approval process but these do not seem to have been well coordinated with the IRBs at the university level. Credentialing is still too complicated with various examinations and refresher courses required for anyone even minimally involved with patient research. Technicians and secretarial staff who may have only the most peripheral involvement with what is going on in terms of the conduct of these studies are required to obtain HIPAA and CITI certification even if they do no more than answer a telephone or schedule an appointment for a patient.

It may seem like petulant nit-picking to complain about any of the regulations that have been put in place. Patient protection and scientific integrity are worthy goals. But even minor additions to the system of controls can eventually add up to an insufferable burden on the individual. A full review of such problems is beyond the scope of this paper but one must express a fear that the growing influence of IRBs and other oversight agencies may well encroach upon the academic freedom of investigators; that talented potential researchers may be discouraged from entering the field in the first place under the weight of such restrictions; and that in the end the very patients the bureaucracy is attempting to protect may be denied the benefits of such important research.

Having grown up professionally in a less regulated clinical research environment during the sixties and seventies I managed to perform my human research ethically relatively unhindered. As the new certifications and recertifications developed within my field of practice and investigation, having been around for so long I usually managed to become "grandfathered" in, without having to meet such requirements. However today, if I had recently entered my field as a cardiologist sub-specializing in echocardiography I would have to look forward to certification and then recertification every seven years in both specialty and sub-specialty cardiology domains. HIPAA and CITI certification also require repeat course work and renewal every three years. The same for cardiopulmonary resuscitation training. The accumulation of a required number of credits in continuing education is required for all hospital staff members in order to maintain staff privileges as well as to remain state licensed. Added to all this in my home state of New Jersey as of April 2008 there is a requirement for attaining "cultural competency." Prior to graduation all medical students must receive specific instruction to this end and all physicians seeking renewal of their licenses must successfully obtain six hours of CME (continuing medical education) credits before approval of their applications.

Meanwhile paper work involved in patient care seems unending and on the increase as well as the resistance of insurers and health maintenance organizations to claims. Along with these operational impediments are continuing threats of litigation in our very litigious society. Patients complain that their doctors do not spend enough time with them. I reply, "How can they?"

IRBs are certainly here to stay. Despite their contribution to the physician-investigators' mounting bureaucratic burden they serve a purpose. Will I remain active now that I have "blown my cover?" Perhaps. As one no longer engaged in the hurly-burly of clinical practice and academic life, I have the time to devote to the task. My continued participation might, in some small way, allow others still with the capacity to extend the boundaries of medical knowledge to meet their patients' needs while, at the same time, pursuing their scientific goals.

REFERENCES

1. Beecher HK. Ethics and Clinical Research. *New Engl J Med* 274:1354-1360, 1966.

2. Rothman DJ. *Strangers at the Bedside: A History of How Law and Bioethics Transformed Medical Decision Making.* (Paperback edition). New York: Aldine de Gruyter, 2003.

3. Weisse AB. *Conversations in Medicine. The story of twentieth century medicine in the words of those who created it.* New York: New York Univ. Press, 1984.

4. Weisse AB. *Heart to Heart. The twentieth century battle against cardiac disease. An oral history.* New Brunswick: Rutgers Univ. Press, 2002.

5. Dunn CM, Chadwick GL. *Protecting study volunteers in research. A manual for investigative sites, 3rd Ed.* Boston: Thomson, 2004.

6. Amdur RJ, Bankert EA. *Institutional review board member handbook, 2nd Ed.* Boston: Jones and Bartlett, 2007.

17

A Skeleton in Obama's Medical Closet: The Doctor Dilemma

AMERICAN MEDICINE CAN JUSTIFIABLY boast of its technological achievements. In few other places in the world can patients obtain the kinds of treatment offered within our borders – provided they have the financial wherewithal to enlist them. It is as a health care delivery system that we have failed miserably. Despite spending one-sixth of our national income on health care, with the highest per capita spending on this in the world, we rank 39th for infant mortality, 43rd for adult female mortality, 42nd for male mortality and 36th for life expectancy compared with other nations in the world.[1] The question has rightly been asked, "Why do we spend so much and get so little?"[2]

The major health care reform bill signed into law by President Obama on May 15, 2010 promises to address many of the health care issues that have bedeviled us. Although it will be two to three years before some of the major provisions of the bill kick in, certain encouraging measures of the most sweeping legislation of this type in decades are becoming apparent already. All Americans will be required by law to obtain health care insurance with over 30 million new subscribers brought under coverage; patients with pre-existing conditions will not be discriminated against by insurers; no caps will be placed on coverage for those who experience catastrophic illnesses with matching costs; children until the age of 26 will be allowed inclusion on their parents' policies; the so-called "donut hole" in Medicare prescription coverage will be eliminated by 2020.

On one point, however, there is general agreement from most experts:

the increasing costs of health care will not be seriously addressed with this legislation. Perhaps if they were the law might not have passed, given the built in obstacles for necessary painful revisions in how we deliver health care.

Beyond such considerations there is another aspect of medical care that has generally remained out of focus: what to do about the doctors. Republican opponents of the health care bill have criticized its neglect of tort reform. The Democrats, in response, have chosen essentially to neglect this aspect of the problem. Yet, whatever health measures go into effect, their chance of achieving success will depend upon the way they are directed through their final route: doctor to patient.

Tort reform, more specifically expressed as the need to address the malpractice problem, is certainly a high priority for any practicing physician. Although over and over again we are reminded that the overwhelming number of complaints against physicians never come to court and among the paltry few that do, rarely does the judgment go against the physician, the possible threat of such a judgment remains a source of high anxiety. Along with this goes the outrageous cost of medical malpractice insurance (converted to increasing fees to patients), and the growing practice of defensive medicine with its hardly insignificant costs to the system. Finally, the litigious nature of much of current medical practice can only serve to further fray the ties of trust between doctor and patient that have characterized this relationship in the past.

What is lost in the rancor of the malpractice debate are other, more subtle influences on how medicine is now being practiced and how much this can further diminish the ability to deliver good health care and erode the intimate doctor-patient relationship itself. What I refer to here are conditions leading to physician "burnout,"the loss of physicians' self-esteem and their mounting resentment against what medical practice has become. Reports of this trend have become commonplace over the last few years. Even in as highly efficient and greatly respected environment as the Mayo Clinic 34 percent of its internists were found to fit into this category.[3] Many physicians are retiring well before their time. Others are cutting back on their services. Many of those still engaged in practice are doing so only to support their families. Is this the kind of personal physician any patient would want to care for him?

One contributing factor to this trend, seemingly unrecognized in Washington, may well be the tendency to emphasize the creation of a *well regulated* contingent of doctors rather than one primarily well motivated and well trained.

Many of the wounds to professional practice are self-inflicted. Over the last several decades a *mea culpa* mind-set has developed among the power brokers of organized medicine supporting the naïve and erroneous idea that any problems with the health care system can be solved by increasing required documentation by physicians that they have the ability to practice intelligently and effectively.[4]

Requirements for certification and periodic recertification for every type of practice have complicated the lives of physicians who wish to remain on staff at hospitals and remain eligible for many group practices. Added to this is certification and recertification under HIPAA (the Health Insurance Portability and Accountability Act) to protect patient privacy. It is certification related to the performance of human research however, in particular, that threatens to stifle such activity on the part of physicians. Permission must be obtained from an IRB (Institutional Review Board) at the hospital and/or medical school affiliate as well as from the granting agency. Before protocols can even be considered by an IRB, CITI (Collaborative Institutional Board Training Initiative) certification must be obtained by the principal investigator, his associates and even his technicians and secretarial staff. Evidence of continuing education efforts, mainly through attendance at conferences and refresher courses, are also required to maintain hospital staff privileges and state licensure. There seems to be no end of ingenuity in devising new putative safeguards against physician malperformance or malfeasance. Recently added to this bureaucratic bundle in my home state of New Jersey is a requirement for attaining "cultural competency" before medical degrees are awarded or state licenses renewed.

It is as if, in an effort to build a protective wall around our patients we have constructed one so thick and daunting that it has become impermeable to the physicians requiring access. Meanwhile physicians are made to feel they are on a never ending treadmill racing after one certification after another just to stay in place. Although we now live in the era of evidence-based medicine it should be noted that none of these programs have ever been critically evaluated for any possible benefits to patient care although persistently poor U.S. health care statistics argue against this. Not surprisingly, in a recent survey among 2500 internists world wide two-thirds of the respondents were found to be against the need for continuing recertification to maintain competence.[5]

Added to all these requirements is the continued burden upon physicians of mounting paper work, reimbursement issues and the aforementioned threat of litigation. The paper work starts early. A recent survey of over 16,000 internal medicine residents revealed that they spend up to twice as much time on documentation as their counterparts did two decades earlier.[6] An equal proportion of respondents revealed that they spent more time on paper work than with patients, some as many as six hours a day. Patients complain that their doctors do not spend enough time with them. With the mounting demands of paper work piling up for them increasingly little time is left for the patients they have dedicated themselves to serve.

Another consideration to be addressed is how current developments in medicine might influence the future supply of physicians. According to a 2005 report of the Council of Graduate Medical Education the number of U.S. physicians will need to grow from 781,000 to as many as 1.2 million by 2020. Most needed will be a supply of primary health care providers. However, the 2009 National Resident Matching Program results indicate that fewer of these positions in primary care (family practice, internal medicine, pediatrics)are being filled than ever in the past. Family Medicine has taken the hardest hit (58 percent of these positions unfilled by American graduating seniors in 2009 compared with 28 percent in 1997).

It is economics that seems to be playing a major role. With an average senior medical student debt of between $130,000 and $140,000 upon graduation, adequate future income to repay these loans is a high priority for those entering the profession. A revealing 1994 study showed a markedly lower yield on educational investment over a working life when primary care physicians were compared with medical specialists as well as business people, dentists and attorneys.[7] A repeat analysis in 2002 again revealed this lower rate of return for primary care physicians.[8] Given such realities it is not surprising that many medical graduates are tending to gravitate toward the higher paying specialties. Although foreign medical graduates can be recruited to make up this deficit, one wonders whether or not this is a wise policy in planning for the future.

Any projected shortage of physicians in the years to come might be exacerbated by working pattern trends among those still listed as actively in practice. The weekly number of hours reported by physicians as devoted to practice is diminishing. Between 1977 and 2007 this fell from and average of almost 56 hours to 51 hours.[9] Five hours a week may not seem like a lot but it is almost ten percent of a physician's time and multiplied by the hundreds of thousands this represents a major decline in the time allotted to patients by their physicians. The recent trend for doctors to abandon their private practices and become hospital employees further reflects their disenchantment with having their own patients for whom they feel primarily responsible. In 2002, 70 percent of practices were privately owned; in 2008 this fell to 50 percent.[10] Accordingly, 50 percent of all medical practices are hospital owned. The institution is replacing the individual as the primary source of medical care.

A final cause for concern is the quality of future students recruited to study medicine. According to data kept by the Association of American Medical Colleges, between 1997 and 2007 the number of applicants to American medical schools has not increased from about 42,000 to 43,000 to keep up with the growth of population. The ratio of applicants to those accepted, about 2.5 to 1.0, has remained constant providing some assurance of selectivity to date. If, however, the number of medical school places increase without a concurrent increase in applicants the admission of those less qualified to be admitted to medical school will certainly increase.

The economic plight of those choosing to study medicine plus the growing number of physician constraints with the likelihood that they will persist can only exacerbate our fears for the future. We must keep in mind that the ultimate effect of any new health legislation will translate into what will transpire between physicians and their patients. Given the current outlook, legitimate concerns can be raised as to whether medicine will continue as an attractive career choice for not only future physicians but for the current cadre of physicians trying to serve their patients either through direct care or through efforts to improve the quality of such care through much needed research into diagnosis and therapy.

We would all welcome the introduction of measures to reduce the current strains on clinical practice and improve the outlook for better medical outcomes by less encumbered physicians engaged either in direct patient care or in related research. However, given the attitudes of the current medical power structure, the glum political landscape in Washington and the overwhelming inertia impeding any effort to undo past errors, no matter how misguided, nothing is likely to happen to change the system until or unless the looming catastrophe is already upon us.

REFERENCES:

1. Doe J. WHO Statistical Information System (WHOSIS) . Geneva. World Health Organization. September 2009.

2. Murray CJL, Frenk J. Ranking 37th – Measuring the performance of the U.S. Health Care System. New Engl J Med 2010;362:96-99.

3. Shanafelt TD, West CP, Sloan JA, Novotny PJ et al. Career fit and burnout among academic faculty. Arch Int Med 2009;169:990-995.

4. Weisse AB. Certification/Recertification: Self-improvement, Self-delusion or Self-strangulation. Persp Biol & Med 1998; 41:579-590.

5. Kritek PA, Drazen JM. American Board of Internal Medicine maintenance of certification program – polling results. New Engl J Med 2010;362:e54.

6. Oxentenko AS, West CP, Popkave C, Weinberger SE, Kolars C. Time spent on clinical documentation: a survey of internal medicine residents and program directors. Arch Int Med 2010;170:377-380.

7. Weeks WB, Wallace AE, Wallace MM, Welch HG, A comparison of educational costs of physicians and other professionals. New Engl J Med 1994;330:1280-1286.

8. Weeks WB, Wallace AE. The more things change: revisiting a comparison of educational costs and incomes of physicians and other professionals. Academic Med 2002;77:313-319.

9. Staiger DO, Auerbach DI, Buerhaus PI. Trends in the work hours of physicians in the United States. JAMA 2010;303:747-753.

10. Harris G, More Doctors Giving Up Private Clinics. NY Times, March 26, 2010.

18

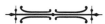

PUBLISHING WITHOUT PERISHING

IT HAS BEEN SAID that every one of us has a least one book in him or her. That being the case, there is none among you who should not be touched by what I have to impart. Of course, whether that book is any good or not is another question and one that can only be answered be your venturing into what I call The Paper Jungle – also known as the World of Publishing. Before I get fully under way I must warn you to expect nothing either morally redeeming or spiritually uplifting from this disclosure. I do hope, however, that you derive a few chuckles along with the nuggets of information I have to offer. I would also like to stress that although my own writing has been primarily medical in nature what I have to relate represents a universality of experience for anyone who has ever considered putting pen to paper.

To begin with, why would anyone want to write a book? According to Samuel Johnson, "No man but a blockhead ever wrote except for money." But if it is money you are after I recommend an honest day job if you hope to keep a roof over your head and put bread on the table. I once read that there were only 100 American authors who were able to support themselves fully through their writing. Now there are over 400 professional players in the National Basketball Association. Statistically, I guess, this means that you have a better chance of playing for the New York Knicks than making it on to the New York Times best seller book list. On the other hand, I have tried to look up precise figures on this and, as best as I can determine, there are over 40,000 new titles in English published each year. You may possibly reassure yourself by thinking, "Well, they've got to publish *someone,* so why not me?"

On the other hand you have to take into account the blockbuster mentality that has overtaken the publishing business. Years ago publishers like Knopf or Random House felt an obligation to promote at least a few promising new authors each year. These were gifted writers whose early works deserved being in print even though the returns to the publisher might be minimal – oftentimes, hopefully, just allowing them to break even. This has gone out of style. Now millions of dollars in advances are given to presumed superstars in hopes of returning more millions to the coffers of the publishers. Bill Clinton, for example, received 12 million dollars in advance for his autobiography. Hillary got 8 million. Charles Frasier, whose best selling novel was *Cold Mountain*, received 8 million in advance for his next work, *13 Moons*. A five book deal earned Mary Higgins Clark 65 million; for two future books Tom Clancy got 45 million in advance. Assume that a struggling full-time writer can subsist on $50,000 for a year; so every million in advances going to some potential heavy hitter precludes the awarding of this lesser sum to 20 deserving writers who lack such notoriety. And an even greater number of other unknown writers who might be able to manage on even less than $50,000 to supplement a small income could also be excluded as a result of such a policy.

What one must also deal with is another facet of the collective psyche of the book publishing industry. Pitch just about any proposal to one of their editors and the response will come in one of two forms: "It's been done already," or "This just cannot be done." And just to pour a little salt into the author's wounds this news will in all likelihood be transmitted through a recent B.A. graduate in English whose only recompense besides sub-standard wages for being employed by a "glamour" industry is the opportunity to stick it to would be authors who can write circles around them

The obtuseness of book editors can further be conveyed by a couple of anecdotes about two prominent authors. The first concerns Doris Lessing and this story I have been able to verify as being true. At a point in her career when she had already been recognized as one of the post-war's pre-eminent writers in English and had been the recipient of a number of literary honors, her agent confirmed to me that she attempted to publish two new works under a pseudonym, Jane Somers. Both were turned down several times by publishing houses and, when finally appearing in hard cover, had only a few reviews and only small print runs. When the truth about the identity of the author was revealed the books were reprinted with her real name and to much acclaim.

The other story concerns the Polish born Jerzy Kosinski. His *The Painted Bird* published in 1965 was hailed as one of the great English language novels of the time. Some intriguing young author got the idea to type up the novel as an original manuscript and send it to Kosinski's publisher under a different name. Not only did the publisher not recognize the work, but it was rejected for its inferior writing. I cannot prove that this is true, but it certainly seems to fit a pattern.

Yet, despite the trials and tribulations of dealing with publishing houses there are people who have absolutely no need to seek them out - those who have achieved all kinds of personal success without them - but who still feel a compulsion to contribute with what might just be the next GREAT AMERICAN NOVEL or its non-fiction equivalent.

I think there is not a better case in point than the cartoonist Charles Schulz. As the creator of the comic strip *Peanuts* he became one of the richest people in America. And even after he died he – or rather those he left behind – continued to rake it in. According to Forbes at one time only Elvis Presley outdid him posthumously. (The income of the estate of the recently deceased Michael Jackson might provide similar competition for earnings beyond the grave.) Schulz's heirs were left with a business empire generating about 1.2 billion dollars in sales annually. During his long career Schulz also received the highest accolades from his fellow cartoonists. He was awarded a Reuben from the National Cartoonists' Society as the outstanding cartoonist in 1955 and again in 1965. But something seemed to be missing.

The most exhaustive writings about Schulz are the authorized biography written by Rheta Johnson in 1989[1] and an even more detailed account by David Michaelis in 2007.[2] In contrast to Schulz's sunny public persona Johnson mentions his neuroses and periods of depression without speculating on their causes and what might have triggered them. Michaelis emphasizes his subject's lifetime love of great literature and mentions Schulz's "yearning for the novelist's life." The connection that both biographies seem to miss emerges in the figure of Snoopy. Although Schulz vigorously denied any reflection of himself in any of his characters to this writer it seems obvious in a number of strips featuring Snoopy as a rejected writer that Schulz, in a humorous way, was conveying his own yearnings along these lines. I reproduce here only three of about a dozen such strips I have saved along the way reflecting this aspect of Schulz (Fig 18.1).

Lacking both the artistic talent and sly humor of Schulz, as an oft-rejected author I was keenly affected by such representations. But it has not been the flurry of rejections greeting my latest creations that has depressed me. I could forgive such misjudgments; there is no accounting for taste; they know not what they do. What I find unconscionable is the all too common practice of holding on to a manuscript with exclusive rights for several months rather than several weeks before choosing to reject the work. Recently I had the

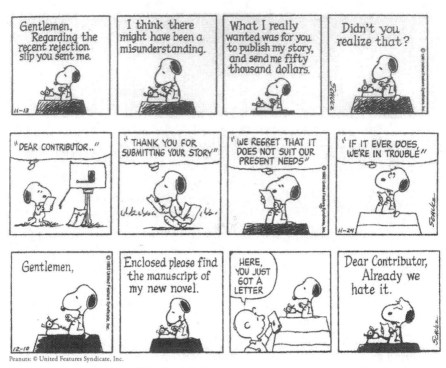

Peanuts: © United Features Syndicate, Inc.

Figure 18.1 Snoopy (Charles Schulz's alter ego) in various throes of authorship (With permission of Peanuts © United Feature Syndicate Inc.)

occasion to send an appropriate response to such behavior. Here is the format with names changed to protect the guilty:

> The Editor
> Lost Horizons Press
> This will confirm that my new book will not be appearing as one of your publications. However, I wish to stress that this in no way need reflect negatively on your professional standing. Given the overwhelming number of competent publishing houses competing for a limited number of superior manuscripts each year, all cannot be accommodated and many worthy institutions such as your own may wind up empty handed. I encourage you not to give up in your efforts.
> The three months during which you were granted exclusive rights to the work, pre-empting offers from any other publishers, might have been considered excessive by some. This extended period might even suggest elements of

laziness or lethargy in the editorial office at Lost Horizons. I prefer to believe that this rather reflects your need to savor and absorb the richness of the prose to which you had been made privy.

Rest assured that you will in no way suffer exclusion from consideration for any new works reaching completion. The door will remain open for any possible future collaboration.

With best wishes for your future success, I remain

Sincerely yours

(Needless to add, I don't believe it would serve any useful purpose to submit any future work to this particular publisher.)

At this point I would like to take you down memory lane with me. I think that many of us who have a desire to see our words in print start early in this quest. My first recorded efforts are still in a collection of scrap books I began in 1945 at the age of 16 when I began to review movies for my George Washington High School classmates in New York City. I continued to pursue my burgeoning career as a critic when I went to New York University up in the Bronx when the University Heights campus was still viable. For the *Heights Daily News* I turned out a different column. It was called "Riding the Airwaves" and covered radio plus the first years of television. I mention these early experiences which included news stories and editorializing from time to time to indicate a learning curve for a tyro journalist. I think it was Hemingway who scoffed at writing schools and said that if anyone wanted to learn to write the only way was just so do it and keep at it in order to improve as with any craft. There certainly is some validity to that view.

In my own case something that I believe may have added to my skills is letter writing – now, with the advent of email and twitter a rapidly dying art. During the two years I was away from home during the Korean War I religiously sent home each week a detailed letter covering not only my personal activities as an Air Force officer but comments on a wide variety of social, political and philosophical issues that concerned me. The collection eventually served as a journal of my time during military service between 1952 and 1954.

The subsequent twenty years of my life as a medical student, house officer and finally academic cardiologist for the most part were not ideal for exercising and improving my skills as an author. Writing medical research papers, incidentally, is the best way of *unlearning* such previously acquired skills that I can imagine with their emphasis on the passive tense and exclusion of the first person singular. But eventually I began turning out non-technical essays and articles. In 1979 I received my first payment for an article I had written. It appeared in *New Jersey Monthly* and recounted my experiences as a dental patient undergoing a major overhaul.[3] It was intended as a humorous piece and described the enormous expense of the undertaking with the wry realization that now, as a doctor who repeatedly unthinkingly ran up enormous debts for his patients without thinking twice about it, I was now receiving my just deserts with the tables turned. The editor substituted *Drilling for Gold* for the original title I proposed and was so pleased with it that he made it the leading article for September 1979. On the cover of the issue there was shown the figure of a chubby physician in obvious need of restorative dental work shaking a finger at the unsuspecting reader. The headline accompanying it in large white print read "A Doctor Speaks Out Against Dentists." Fortunately my name was not revealed as the source of such a misleading slant on my work especially in the light of the unintended consequences of this inadvertently inflammatory piece of journalism. Although the two dentists who were working to restore my choppers joined me in amusement about the piece, they were apparently the only two dentists in the state of New Jersey who did. Every other dentist seemed to be outraged by the article and since most of them subscribed to *New Jersey Monthly* for their waiting rooms this represented an important source of income for the magazine. As a result of the massive cancellation of subscriptions that ensued the magazine went out of business a few months later thanks to my sterling contribution. I apologized to the editor for putting him and his staff out of work but he stuck by his guns in supporting me. Fortunately there is a new *New Jersey Monthly* back in operation as of the last few years so there is some consolation in this. Despite this early mishap I never gave up on writing articles for medical and other periodicals. It was these small boosts to my ego that kept me going and eventually organizing them in book form.

My big break came in 1984 thanks to a friend and mentor, Charles Mangel, a successful professional writer and former editor at *Look* magazine. He had a contract to do a popular book on medical advances and needed help in fulfilling it. He made me co-author of what became *Medicine: State of the Art*.[4] I was now a published author. It turned out that in the same year I got a series of interviews with outstanding medical figures published by New York University Press. It was called *Conversations in Medicine* and proved an auspicious beginning.[5] *Conversations'* sales were between five and six thousand copies and the book also received an award from *Library Journal* as one of the 100 best books in science for 1984. At the same time, however, it was the experience with NYU Press that first revealed to me how lame or misleading many university presses may be when it comes to marketing, which is critical for the commercial success of any book. NYU had initially provided me with an extensive list of all the marketing ploys they intended to employ in making the book succeed, including advertising in choice outlets.

With over five thousand copies sold I had hopes for even greater sales resulting from the slam bang campaign that I thought would swing into action. When I asked the editor when this would all take place he exploded. In a scathing letter he chided me for expecting any such action before the sales of the book warranted it. Funny, I had always thought that you advertised to bring on the sales and not the other way around. The fact is that almost all university presses are underfunded for such activities and it is naïve for any author working for them to expect anything approaching a meaningful marketing campaign for their books.

Something else that might do the trick is a good review in a periodical like the *New Yorker Magazine* or the *New York Times*. However, with perhaps 40 or 50 thousand new books coming down the line each year and the capability of such publications to handle only a small fraction of them, the chances of your own book – without any significant marketing – of getting reviewed are minimal to non-existent. And if you do get reviewed there is no guarantee that the review will be good. I have entertained the fantasy of being reviewed my Michiko Kakutani of the *New York Times* one day. She is about as prominent a critic as you could wish for but is probably the most adept one at slipping the proverbial knife between the ribs of hapless authors. Ms Kakutani is also capable of writing favorable reviews but they seem few and far between.

With my first two books in print I was able to attract the attention of an agent who did me one good turn by getting me a contract with *Consumers Reports Books* to do a book on male health.[6] I took it on as a challenge requiring my covering many areas of medicine with which I was not readily conversant rather than something I really enjoyed doing. I made some money and was pleased to find that I was the single author for the male book while *Consumers' Reports* needed four women, I believe, to do the companion book for the ladies. Fortunately I had a full-time day job and I was never tempted into a similar arrangement, attractive only financially as lucrative as that might be.

My agent failed to find anything else for me over the next few years and I eventually decided to look for publishing possibilities on my own. Perhaps this is a good point at which to mention vanity presses. They offer to print your book and the cost for a few hundred copies is not outrageous. But for me there are two possible reasons against going this route. First of all, even though I am not seeking to become rich as the primary reward for my efforts, I look upon it as an important matter of self-esteem to have someone else think my work worthy enough to invest in publishing it. Second, once the copies of your book are handed over to you by the vanity press you become the distributor of the book and have to pay for your own marketing. And who knows knows anything about that? You are even worse off than you would have otherwise been with a university press as limited as their marketing funds are.

For my next few books I pretty much stuck with university presses. Rutgers handled *Medical Odysseys,* a book about how medical discoveries are made.[7] The University of Southern Illinois Press published *The Staff and the Serpent,* a collection of essays on medicine described as either pertinent or impertinent.[8] I returned to Rutgers in my home state for *Heart to Heart,* another oral history, this one tapping the life stories of outstanding figures in cardiology and cardiovascular surgery.[9]

Despite my growing recognition as a medical writer none of these books, to the best of my knowledge, ever came close to the five thousand plus sales of *Conversations in Medicine.* However, I could live with this. What I did find hard to tolerate were comments from friends soon to become ex-friends who would sidle up to me at medical meetings and say, "I saw your book on sale at Barnes and Noble yesterday. It was only a dollar." Or inform me that they had checked on my book sales at Amazon.com and discovered that I was number 169,355 in sales. I didn't know they even counted that high (or, more accurately, that low) for the rankings and I certainly was not interested in finding out about it.

It was not that I totally accepted this sad situation about my book sales and I tried to do whatever little I could on my own to stimulate them. Once it was suggested to me that I have a book signing at the local Barnes and Noble. At the time of my appearance as I sat down at the end of an aisle at the back of the store I was joined by my wife and mother-in-law. The only other human to appear was an elderly lady who had stumbled across us while looking for the Geography Section. It was one of the most humiliating experiences of my writer's life. Well, perhaps not the *most* humiliating. Six months after the appearance of one of my books I checked with marketing to learn how well it was doing. It had sold 750 copies, which seemed encouraging to the party at the other end of the line. With future expectations like sugar plums dancing in my head I waited until another six months had passed before making another inquiry. I was informed that the annual sales had now reached 725. "How could this be?" I asked incredulously. Simple mathematics: 25 copies had been returned without the sale of a single additional copy.

So how do you become a rich and famous writer? Well, famous anyway. Winning a Nobel Prize in Literature would be one way. It seemed to work for Elfriede Jelinek a couple of years ago. Just before her being anointed her novel *The Piano Teacher* was 1,163,804 on the Amazon sales ranking list. I'm sure the Nobel boosted it a few hundred thousand at least. But I certainly was not in line for a Nobel or any other prize for that matter.

One of my friends said that what I would have to do is write a best seller.

"What do you have in mind?" I asked. He explained to me that there are three genres of books that always sell well: books about Lincoln; books about doctors; and books about dogs. The obvious solution was to write a book entitled "Lincoln's Doctor's Dog." Although I could not work up enough enthusiasm to embark on this route I did believe I could at least turn out a novel about a doctor.

The title was to be "The Case," and I actually managed to produce some sample chapters for various accommodating victims to peruse. I gave the story a medical background and it was to be a roman à clef. The leading character was me, in literary drag as an overweight young Jewish woman working as a medical resident in a high powered teaching hospital. Her husband is a ne'er do well WASP type whom she eventually sheds. The case referred to in the title is one of malpractice brought against our heroine and of course she is entirely innocent. After many ups and downs in the plot she is finally vindicated. She rejects the choice research position offered her at the university and rides off into the sunset in the direction of an Indian reservation overflowing with adorable tubercular kiddies needing her attention. It was awful. I hated the idea and it showed. My roman à clef was turning out to be a roman à clunk. I soon dropped it and never again ventured upon a subject about which I was not completely enthusiastic.

This brings me to my most recently published work, *Lessons in Mortality.*[10] It is a collection of true stories about patients and doctors facing disease, death and one another. I felt it was a book with a good deal of human interest, minimal technical detail, and a natural for the general public. It turned out to be the most difficult sell of my career but I was not to be denied.

I recalled the story of John H. Johnson who rose from humble circumstances to become head of a corporate empire that included *Ebony* magazine, a major cosmetic company and many other enterprises. I was listening to an interview he granted over public radio some years ago when he was asked about the major key to his success. His reply was "Persistence." He recalled as an example how he had wanted an interview with Eleanor Roosevelt for his magazine and how she had turned him down five times before granting it after a sixth request. So I made persistence my guiding principle.

I began with contacting 20 trade publishers but none of them were interested. Most informed me that they would not even consider a manuscript unless it had been handed in by a literary agent. If an agent was what I needed to break down the literary barriers then so be it. In search of a new agent I contacted 160 over a six year period. About one in ten offered to look at the manuscript; none of them expressed an interest in pursuing the matter further.

As I struggled to gain representation I gradually became convinced that a university press, after all, might be my only hope for seeing the book in print. I obtained a copy of *Literary Market Place* an annual publication the size of the Manhattan telephone directory that lists every publishing house, agent etc. in the field. This provided me with the names of the editors and addresses of every university press in the country. But to which ones should I send a proposal? I had already unsuccessfully sounded out and been rejected by about a half dozen of them noted for publishing medical history and related topics. I simply began with the beginning of the alphabet, contacting all presses with at least 30 books to their credit each year in order to maximize my chances. I had just finished working my way through the m's when a letter arrived from the University of Missouri Press expressing interest. The book was published in 2006 and they did a fine job. The editor-in-chief became a fan of mine and kept asking me for my next literary gem. However when it was finally nearing completion and I was ready to send in what I had completed I learned that my favorite editor had retired. Her successor took a look and turned it down. And so it goes. There may come a point at which there is not even a university press that will come to your rescue. It was at this point that I decided to self-publish with iUniverse. By choosing to go this route, I am at least assured of having my book between hard (or soft) covers, listed with the Library of Congress and available on demand from Amazon and other book dealers.

Above all you must keep the faith. Aside from enthusiasm for your own work, your belief in it and your persistence in promoting it, it helps to remember how many writers with much greater gifts than you have suffered rejection. Some years ago a short piece appeared in the New York Times Book Review entitled "We're Sorry, but…" It was a review of a book entitled *Rejection* by John White. I framed it and occasionally re-read it during the tough times of my own rejections.

Among the sobering facts included is one involving James Joyce whose *Dubliners* was rejected by 22 publishers. When at last it was accepted for publication someone bought out the entire run that had been printed and had it burned in Dublin. James M. Caine, it was reported, titled his novel *The Postman Always Rings Twice* because it had been rejected so many times before publication that each day the postman had to ring twice to handle all the bad news. Giuseppi di Lampedusa was so distraught over a publisher's rejection of the only book he ever wrote that he hid the manuscript and died thinking his life's work was worthless. But *The Leopard* became a posthumous great success on both sides of the Atlantic. Beatrix Potter's perennial *best* seller, *The Tale of Peter Rabbit,"* was rejected by at least seven publishers. It was not until the author published it herself that Frederick Warne, one of the the seven, changed his mind and agreed to take it on.

Other outstanding books reportedly rejected at least once by Mr. White are *War and Peace, Lust for Life, The Good Earth, The Fountainhead, To Kill a Mockingbird* and *A Confederacy of Dunces.*

Oscar Wilde had priceless rejoinders for just about everything. One of them is particularly germane to the subject at hand. The night before the opening of one of his plays – *The Importance of Being Ernest,* I believe – he was asked if he thought it would be a success. "Oh the play is already a success," he replied. "The question is will the audience be a success?" That's the kind of attitude we struggling authors need to cultivate. Like Oscar you must learn to scoff at rejection and giggle at adversity.

There is a quasi-existentialist question that is often put: If a tree falls in the forest and there is no one there to witness it does it make a sound? A similar type of question might be put to the creative writer: If you were the only person in the world and there was no other person existing who could read what you have written would you continue to write? In this context it is J.D. Salinger who comes most readily to mind. Widely heralded as one of the greatest new American novelists of his time after the appearance of "Catcher in the Rye"(1951) and other works, Salinger decidedly rejected the notoriety that attended this. In 1953 he moved to Cornish, New Hampshire, and began the life of a recluse that ended only with his death in 2010 at the age of 91. His last publication was a story that appeared in the New Yorker Magazine in 1965. In 1974 during a rare interview granted he was quoted , "But I write just for myself and my own pleasure." He reiterated his opinion of the publishing business as "a terrible invasion of privacy." If such was the case we might have expected a treasure load of material that had been squirreled away in his cabin over the years, but nothing was found at the time of his death.

Whether one writes for himself or others is a tough question to answer for anyone hoping to enrich the intellectual and emotional life of others by the product of his pen. For me it becomes easier to reply if I were told that there was still one person left in the world other than myself who might be able to read what I have written. I can respond to this with an anecdote.

Over twenty years ago when *Conversations in Medicine* was published one of those interviewed for the book was Marian Ropes, a pioneer rheumatologist at the Massachusetts General Hospital where she was the first female medical resident in its hundred year history. She became a role model for later generations of women physicians. At the time of her death many years after the book had appeared I received a letter from one of her family members in which I was informed that at the funeral it was quotes from my extended interview with her that constituted the bulk of the memorial service. Recalled in this way, her actual spoken words brought her spirit that much closer to all who attended. I was thanked for making this possible. Even if this gentleman was the only person in the world to have read the book it would still have been worth everything.

REFERENCES

1. Johnson RG. *Good Grief: The Story of Charles M. Schulz.* New York: Pharos Books, 1989.

2. Michaelis D. *Schulz and Peanuts.* New York: Harper Collins, 2007.

3. Physician JQ. Drilling for Gold. An Odyssey through the world of oral surgery, reconstruction and high finance. *New Jersey Monthly* 1979;Sept: 55-57.

4. Mangel C, Weisse AB. *Medicine: The State of the Art.* New York: Dial Press, 1984.

5. Weisse AB. *Conversations in Medicine. The Story of 20th Century Medicine in the Words of Those Who Created It.* New York: New York Univ. Press, 1984.

6. Weisse AB. *The Man's Guide to Good Health.* New York: Consumers Reports Books, 1991.

7. Weisse AB. *Medical Odysseys. The Different and Sometimes Unexpected Pathways to 20th Century Medical Discoveries.* New Brunswick: Rutgers Univ. Press, 1991.

8. Weisse AB. *The Staff and the Serpent. Pertinent and Impertinent Observations on the World of Medicine.* Carbondale: Southern Illinois Univ. Press, 1998.

9. Weisse AB. *Heart to Heart. The Twentieth Century Battle Against Cardiac Disease. An Oral History.* New Brunswick: Rutgers Univ. Press, 2002.

10. Weisse AB. *Lessons in Mortality. Doctors and Patients Struggling Together.* Columbia & London: Univ. of Missouri Press, 2006.

About the Author:
Allen B. Weisse, M.D.

With over 40 years as a cardiologist, professor of medicine, researcher, historian and keen observer of the medical scene, Dr. Weisse has forged a career as both a chronicler and critic of his chosen profession.

His career in academic medicine has produced over a hundred professional publications. His abiding interest in the history of medicine and medicine's current place in society led to his first books, *Medicine: State of the Art* (Dial) in 1984 and the award-winning *Conversations in Medicine* (NYU Press) in the same year. In 1991 his continued interest in the progress of cardiovascular and other health research produced *Medical Odysseys: The Different and Sometimes Unexpected Pathways of 20th Century Medical Discoveries* (Rutgers University Press). His concern with promoting personal health was reflected in *The Man's Guide to Good Health* (Consumer Reports Books), also appearing in 1991. He has been a frequent contributor to various magazines and a collection of essays, *The Staff and the Serpent: Pertinent and Impertinent Observations on the World of Medicine* (Southern Illinois University Press), appeared in 1998. *Heart to Heart. The Twentieth Century Battle Against Cardiac Disease. An Oral History*, published by Rutgers University Press, appeared in 2002. His latest work, a collection of medical stories entitled *Lessons in Mortality: Doctors and Patients Struggling Together* (University of Missouri Press) appeared in 2006.

He has been a member of the American Heart Association for over 40 years and is board-certified in Internal Medicine and Cardiovascular Diseases. He has been a fellow of the American College of Cardiology since 1968. A recent past president of the Medical History Society of New Jersey and a member of the American Association for the History of Medicine and the American Osler Society, he lectures frequently throughout the country on a variety of subjects related to medical history and ethics as well as cardiovascular disease.

In 1997, in order to devote himself more fully to his writing and historical interests, he resigned his full-time position as Professor of Medicine at the New Jersey Medical School although he remains on the faculty as a clinical professor, stimulating new generations of students and house officers to explore the past and move knowledgeably into the future of American medicine. The Weisse Lecture on the History of Medicine was endowed as an annual event at the New Jersey Medical School in 2004.